Gurteshwar Singh

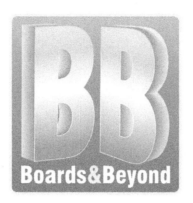

Boards and Beyond: Cardiology Slides

Slides from the Boards and Beyond Website

Jason Ryan, MD, MPH

2019 Edition

Table of Contents

Cardiac Anatomy	1	Heart Murmurs	96
Cardiac Physiology	3	Heart Sounds	101
CV Response to Exercise	8	Heart Failure Basics	105
Blood Flow Mechanics	10	Systolic and Diastolic Heart Failure	111
Regulation of Blood Pressure	16	Restrictive Cardiomyopathy	115
PV Loops	20	Acute Heart Failure	118
Wiggers' Diagram	24	Chronic Heart Failure	123
Venous Pressure Tracings	26	Cardiac Embryology	127
Starling Curve	28	Shunts	131
Atherosclerosis	31	Cyanotic Congenital Heart Disease	135
Cardiac Ischemia	35	Coarctation of the Aorta	141
STEMI	42	Hypertension	145
Unstable Angina/NSTEMI	47	Secondary Hypertension	148
Stable angina	49	Hypertension drugs	153
EKG Basics	55	Valve Disease	161
High Yield EKGs	61	Shock	167
Action Potentials	65	Pericardial Disease	171
AV and Bundle Branch Blocks	69	Aortic dissection	177
Atrial Fibrillation	74	Cardiac Tumors	181
AVNRT	81	Hypertrophic Cardiomyopathy	184
WPW	83	Endocarditis	188
Antiarrhythmic Drugs	85		

Lungs → Pulmonary vein → LA → LV

Cardiac Anatomy
Jason Ryan, MD, MPH

The Heart
Chambers

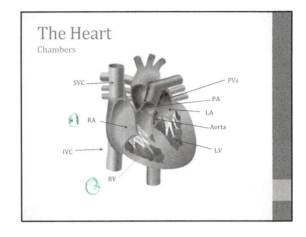

Labels: SVC, RA, IVC, RV, PVs, PA, LA, Aorta, LV

The Heart
Valves

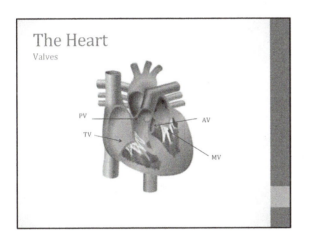

Labels: PV, TV, AV, MV

Right ventricle is Ant to chest

Anterior-Posterior Structures

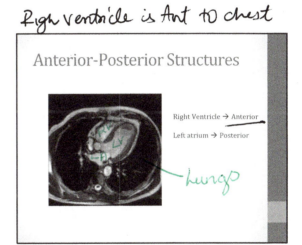

Right Ventricle → Anterior
Left atrium → Posterior

Lungs

Coronary Arteries

90% Right dominant
10% Left dominant

Heart drains to coronary sinus
CS → Right atrium

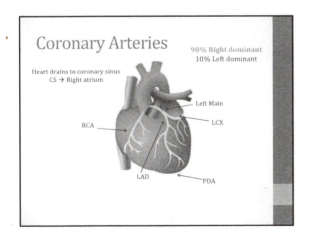

Labels: RCA, Left Main, LCX, LAD, PDA

Coronary Artery Territories

- Anterior wall, anterior septum, apex → LAD
- Lateral wall → LCX
- Inferior wall, inferior septum → PDA
  - RCA 90% of the time
  - 10% of people "left dominant" - LCX supplies PDA
- Occlusion occurs LAD>RCA>LCX

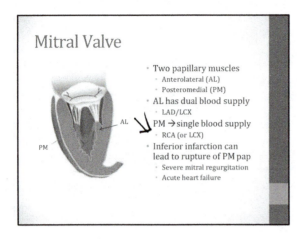

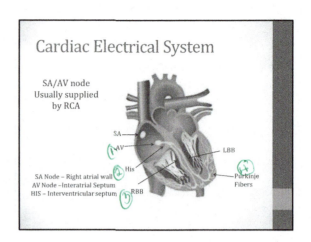

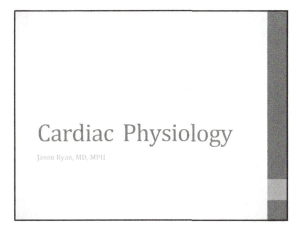

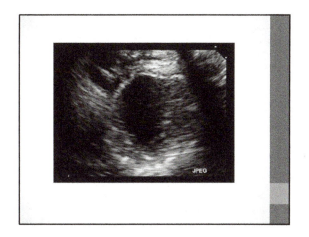

ESV: volume at end of systole

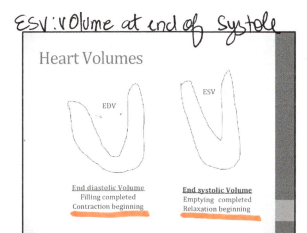

Important Terms

- Stroke Volume (SV) = EDV − ESV
- Ejection Fraction (EF) = SV / EDV — % of blood pushed out LV
- Cardiac Output (CO) = SV * HR

Important Terms

- Venous Return (VR)
  - Blood returned to left ventricle
  - Should be equal to the cardiac output
- Total peripheral resistance
  - Resistance to blood flow from peripheral structures
  - Vasoconstriction → ↑ TPR
  - Vasodilation → ↓ TPR

Blood Pressure Terms

- Systolic Blood Pressure (SBP)
  - Largely determined by stroke volume
- Diastolic Blood Pressure (DBP)
  - Largely determined by TPR
- Pulse pressure
  - SBP − DBP
  - Proportional to SV

Blood Pressure Terms

- **Mean arterial pressure (MAP)**
  - DBP + 1/3 (SBP – DBP)
- Example: SBP 120/80
  - MAP = 80 + 1/3 (40) = 93.3

Cardiac Output

- Very important physiology parameter
- Must rise to meet demands
- More cardiac output = more work/O2
  - CO = HR x SV
  - More beats per minute = more work
  - More volume per beat = more work

Cardiac Output
Determinants

1. Preload
2. Afterload
3. Contractility
4. Heart rate

Preload

- Amount of blood loaded into left ventricle
- Also how much stretch is on fibers prior to contraction
  - Some books say "length" instead of "stretch"
- More preload = more cardiac output
- More preload = more work the heart must do
  - ↑O$_2$ required

To INCREASE Preload

1. Add volume (blood, IVF)
2. Slow heart rate → more filling → more volume
3. Constrict veins
   - Veins force blood into heart
   - Veins hold LARGE blood volume
   - Response to blood loss → venous constriction
   - Sympathetic stimulation → α1 receptors in veins

To DECREASE Preload

1. Remove volume (bleeding, dehydration)
2. Raise heart rate (opposite mechanism above)
3. Pool blood in veins
   - Mechanism of action of nitrates
   - Relieve angina
   - Lower preload → less work for heart

Preload
Important Terms

- LVEDV
  - Volume of blood in the left ventricle when filled
- LVEDP
  - Pressure in the left ventricle when filled

Afterload

- Forces resisting flow out of left ventricle
- Heart must squeeze to increase pressure
- Needs to open aortic valve → push blood into aorta
- This is harder to do if:
  - Blood pressure is high
  - Aortic valve is stiff
  - Something in the way: HCM, sub-aortic membrane

To INCREASE Afterload

1. Raise mean blood pressure MBP
2. Obstruct outflow of left ventricle
   - Aortic stenosis, HCM

To DECREASE Afterload

1. Lower the mean blood pressure
2. Treat aortic valve disease, HCM
- More afterload = more work
  - More oxygen required

Contractility

- How hard the heart muscle squeezes
- Ejection fraction = index of contractility
- Major regulator: **sympathetic nervous system**
  - Also increases heart rate

To INCREASE Contractility

- Sympathetic nervous system activity
  - Sympathetic innervation to heart
  - Circulating catecholamines (epinephrine, norepinephrine)
  - ↑ calcium release from sarcoplasmic reticulum
  - Triggers: stress, exercise
- Sympathomimetic drugs
  - Dopamine, dobutamine, epinephrine, norepinephrine
- Digoxin
  - Inhibits Na-K pump → ↑ calcium in myocytes

To DECREASE Contractility

- Sympathetic system blocking drugs
  - Beta blockers
- Calcium channel blockers
  - Verapamil, diltiazem
  - Less calcium for muscle contraction
- Heart failure
  - Disease of myocytes

Heart Rate

- Increases cardiac output under physiologic conditions
- Mainly regulated by sympathetic nervous system
- Also increased by **sympathomimetic drugs**
- Decreased by beta blockers and calcium blockers

Heart Rate

- ↑ HR = ↓ stroke volume (less filling time)

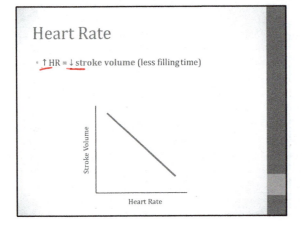

Heart Rate

- ↑HR = ↑ cardiac output

CO = SV * HR

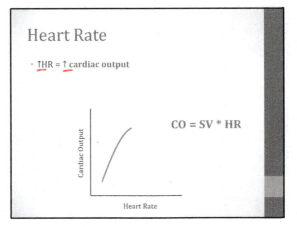

Heart Rate

- Sympathetic nervous system: ↑HR and ↑contractility
- Stroke volume rises with increased HR

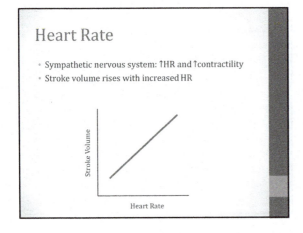

Heart Rate

- At pathologic heart rates ↑ HR = ↓ CO
- High heart rate with arrhythmia can lead to ↓CO

↓CO = ↓SV * HR↑

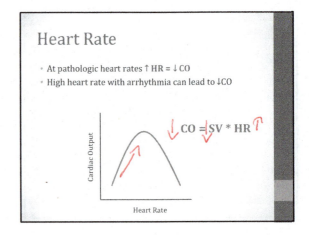

Work of the heart
Myocardial O2 demand

- Preload (LVEDV/P)
- Afterload (MAP)
- Contractility (EF)
- Heart Rate

Hearts starved for O2 → Reduce O2 demand
Low output → Need to increase work

Cardiovascular Response to Exercise

Jason Ryan, MD, MPH

Response to Exercise

- Body's overall goal:
  - Maximize perfusion skeletal muscles and heart
  - Minimize perfusion all other areas
- Initiator: **Muscle hypoxia**
- Mediator: **Sympathetic nervous system**

Response to Exercise

- Process begins with muscle contraction
- ATP consumed → oxygen consumed (need more ATP)
- Result: Local hypoxia in muscle tissue
- Vasodilation occurs
  - Multiple mediators released into plasma
  - Adenosine generated from ATP consumption
  - Lactate
  - Carbon dioxide, potassium
- **Lowers total peripheral resistance (TPR)**

Response to Exercise

- **Sympathetic nervous system** activated
- ↑contractility (stroke volume)
- ↑HR
- Net result: ↑ cardiac output
- Results in ↑ **systolic blood pressure (SBP)**
- Vasoconstriction in some areas (gut, skin)
  - Redistributes blood to important areas (i.e. heart/muscles)

Response to Exercise
Blood Pressure Summary

- SBP rises
  - More CO = more blood in arteries = more pressure
  - Primary determinant systolic BP = cardiac output
- DBP decreases slightly or stays normal
  - Local dilation of skeletal muscles
  - Primary determinant diastolic BP = peripheral resistance
- Pulse pressure increases
- TPR goes down

Response to Exercise
Ejection Fraction

$$EF = \frac{EDV - ESV}{EDV}$$

- LVEF increases
  - More vigorous contraction
  - Major impact: ESV decreases
  - EDV effects minor/variable
  - More preload but less filling time at fast heart rates

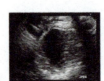 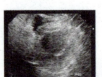

Response to Exercise
Coronary Perfusion

- Fast HR shortens diastole
- LESS coronary filling time
- Coronary vasodilation → increased blood flow
  - Only way to get more oxygen
  - Cannot extract more O_2
  - Cardiac tissue extracts maximum oxygen from RBCs
  - Cannot extract more to meet increased demand

Response to Exercise
Preload

- Preload rises with exercise
- Sympathetic stimulation → **venous contraction**
- Increases preload/EDV
- Contributes to rise in cardiac output
  - Along with increased heart rate and contractility

Lusitropy

- Lusitropy = **myocardial relaxation**
  - Opposite of contractility
- Increased with exercise
- Contributes to increased preload → ↑ cardiac output

Lusitropy

- Key regulatory protein: Phospholamban
  - Inhibitor: sarcoplasmic reticulum Ca2+-ATPase (SERCA)
  - Phosphorylated via beta adrenergic stimulation
  - Stops inhibiting SERCA
  - Result: SERCA takes up calcium → relaxation

SERCA
Sarco/endoplasmic reticulum Ca^{2+}-ATPase

- Sympathetic stimulation → phosphorylates PLB
- Inactivates PLB (relieves inhibitory effect)
- Allows SERCA to uptake more calcium

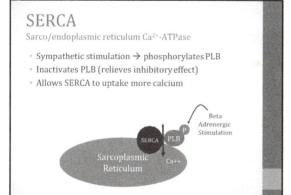

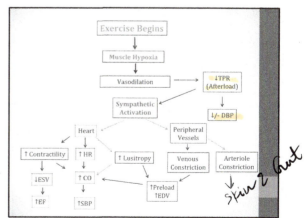

- Exercise → ATP (O_2) consumed → Muscle hypoxia → Vasodilators released → decrease TPR (↓ Diastolic BP) → Sympathic nervous system activated

Fluids:- driving force is the pressure change = ΔP

Blood Flow Mechanics

Jason Ryan, MD, MPH

Flow Equations

Ohm's Law $V = IR$ For fluids: $\Delta P = Q \times R$ $CO = Q$ for body TPR = total peripheral resistance
$\Delta P = CO \times TPR$

Flow Equations

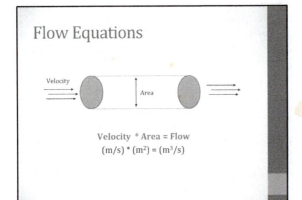

Velocity * Area = Flow
$(m/s) * (m^2) = (m^3/s)$

Resistance and Compliance

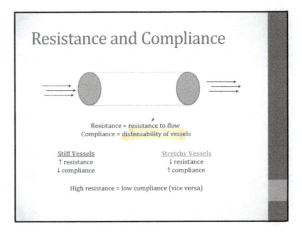

Resistance = resistance to flow
Compliance = distensability of vessels

Stiff Vessels
↑ resistance
↓ compliance

Stretchy Vessels
↓ resistance
↑ compliance

High resistance = low compliance (vice versa)

Pulse Pressure

- Systolic BP – diastolic BP
  - Normal = 120 – 80 = 40mmHg
- Older patients = ↑ pulse pressure
- Hypertensive patients = ↑ pulse pressure
- Related to **vessel compliance**
- ↓ compliance = ↑ pulse pressure

Pulse Pressure

- Compliance = Δ volume / Δ pressure
- Stiff vessel → ↓ compliance → ↑ pulse pressure
  - Small change in volume for given pressure applied to walls
- Stretchy vessel → ↑ compliance → ↓ pulse pressure
  - Large change in volume for given pressure applied to walls

$$C = \Delta V / \Delta P$$
$$\downarrow$$
$$\Delta P = \Delta V / C$$

Fluids:- driving force is the pressure change = ΔP

Pulse Pressure

- Pulse pressure varies with vessel compliance
- Stiff vessels → ↓ compliance

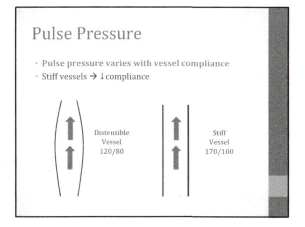

Distensible Vessel 120/80

Stiff Vessel 170/100

Flow Equation
Total Peripheral Resistance

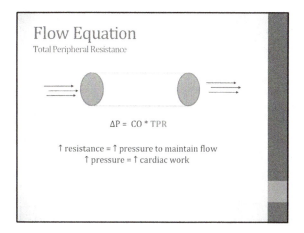

$$\Delta P = CO * TPR$$

↑ resistance = ↑ pressure to maintain flow
↑ pressure = ↑ cardiac work

Total Peripheral Resistance

- Easy to push blood out of heart → less O_2 required
- Resistance to flow → more work for heart
- What resists forward flow out of heart?
  1. Types of vessels (i.e. pipes/tubes)
  2. Thickness of blood (viscosity)

Types of Vessels

- Aorta: SBP 100mmHg
- Large arteries: Falls few mmHg
- Small arteries: 10-20mmHg
- Arterioles: 35mmHg
- Capillaries: 25mmHg

Types of Vessels

- Arterioles = "resistance vessels"
  - Major determinant of total peripheral resistance
  - Large pressure drop
  - Vasoconstriction = ↑ TPR
  - Vasodilation = ↓ TPR

Viscosity

- Thickness of blood
- Low viscosity
  - Anemia
- High viscosity
  - Polycythemia
  - Multiple myeloma
  - Spherocytosis

Poiseuille's Law

- $\Delta P = Q \times R$

$$R = \frac{\Delta P}{Q} = \frac{8\eta \text{ (viscosity) } L \text{ (length)}}{\Pi r \text{ (radius)}^4}$$

Changes in radius → large change in resistance

[handwritten note: resistance ↑ when viscosity goes up]

Series and Parallel Circuits

Human organs arranged in parallel
Resistances add up differently in series than in parallel

$$\frac{1}{R_{total}} = \frac{1}{R_1} + \frac{1}{R_2} \qquad R_{total} = R_1 + R_2$$

Parallel   Series

Series and Parallel Circuits

For two resistances (2 and 2), what is total R?

$$\frac{1}{R_{total}} = \frac{1}{R_1} + \frac{1}{R_2} \qquad R_{total} = R_1 + R_2$$
$$R_{total} = 2 + 2 = 4$$

$$\frac{1}{R_{total}} = \frac{1}{2} + \frac{1}{2}$$

$R_{total} = 1$

Flow Equation $\Delta P = Q * R$

- Used to calculate resistance, CO, or ΔP
- Often applied to body and lungs
  - For both systems Q = Cardiac Output (CO)

Flow Equation $\Delta P = Q * R$

- Body
  - ΔP = Arterial pressure – right atrial pressure
  - R = Total peripheral resistance (TPR)
  - R = Systemic vascular resistance (SVR)
- Lungs
  - ΔP = Pulmonary artery pressure – left atrial pressure
  - R = Pulmonary vascular resistance (PVR)

Mean Arterial Pressure

- Diastolic plus 1/3 (Systolic – Diastolic)
- Total body
  - Arterial blood pressure = 120/80 mmHg
  - Mean arterial pressure = 80 + 1/3 (40) = 93 mmHg
- Lungs
  - Pulmonary artery pressure = 40/20 mmHg
  - Mean pulmonary artery pressure = 20 + 1/3 (20) = 27 mmHg

Total Body

$$\Delta P = CO * TPR$$

- R = TPR
- ΔP = MAP − RAP
  - MAP = mean arterial pressure
  - RAP = right atrial pressure
- CO of 5L/min; BP 155/80 (MAP 105), RA 5

$$TPR = \frac{\Delta P}{CO} = \frac{MAP - RAP}{5} = \frac{105 - 5}{5} = 20$$

Lungs

$$\Delta P = CO * TPR$$

- R = PVR
- ΔP = PA − LAP
  - PA = mean pulmonary artery pressure
  - LAP = left atrial pressure
- CO of 5L/min; PA 40/10 (MAP 20), LA 5

$$PVR = \frac{\Delta P}{CO} = \frac{PA - LAP}{5} = \frac{20 - 5}{5} = 3$$

Lung and Body Flow Variables

	Lung	Body
Flow	CO	CO
Resistance	PVR	TPR
Start Pressure	PA	AoP
End Pressure	LA	RA
ΔP	PA − LA	Ao − RA

Velocity and Area

- Flow = Velocity * Area
- Changes as blood moves through vessels
  - Aorta → arterioles → capillaries → veins
  - Cardiac output moves through system (same flow)
  - Different vessels → different area, velocity
  - Area ↑↑, velocity ↓↓

Flow = Velocity * Area
$(m^3/s) = (m/s) * (m^2)$

Flow Properties of Blood Vessels

Property	Highest	Lowest
Flow	--	--
Area	Capillaries	Large arteries
Velocity	Large Arteries	Capillaries
Resistance	Arterioles	Veins
ΔP	Arterioles	Veins

Flow = Vel * Area
$\Delta P = Q \times R$

Law of Laplace

- Wall tension or wall stress
- Applies to vessels and cardiac chambers
- ↑ tension → ↑ O2 demand → ischemia/angina

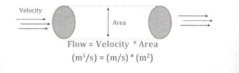

$$Tension \propto \frac{P * r}{2h}$$

Wall Tension

- Afterload: Increases **pressure** in left ventricle
  - Hypertension, aortic stenosis
  - Will increase wall tension
  - "Pressure overload"

$$\text{Tension} \propto \frac{P * r}{2h}$$

Wall Tension

- Preload: Increases **radius** of left ventricle
  - Chronic valvular disease (aortic/mitral regurgitation)
  - Will increase wall tension
  - "Volume overload"

$$\text{Tension} \propto \frac{P * r}{2h}$$

Wall Tension

- Hypertrophy: Compensatory mechanism
  - Will decrease wall tension
  - Force distributed over more mass
  - Occurs with chronic pressure/volume overload

$$\text{Tension} \propto \frac{P * r}{2h}$$

Eccentric Hypertrophy

- Longer myocytes
- Sarcomeres added in series
- Left ventricular mass increased
- Wall thickness NOT increased

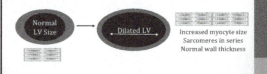

Normal LV Size → Dilated LV

Increased myocyte size
Sarcomeres in series
Normal wall thickness

Eccentric Hypertrophy

- **Volume overload of left ventricle**
  - Aortic regurgitation
  - Mitral regurgitation
- Cardiomyopathy
  - Ischemic and non-ischemic

Concentric Hypertrophy

- Pressure overload
- Chronic ↑↑ pressure in ventricle
- Sarcomeres added in parallel
- Left ventricular mass increased
- Wall thickness increased

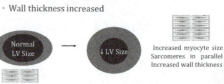

Normal LV Size → ↓ LV Size

Increased myocyte size
Sarcomeres in parallel
Increased wall thickness

Concentric Hypertrophy

- Classic causes: Hypertension, Aortic stenosis
  - Both raise pressure in LV cavity
- Decreased compliance (stiff ventricle)
- Often seen in diastolic heart failure

Regulation of Blood Pressure

Jason Ryan, MD, MPH

Blood Pressure

- Required for perfusion of tissues
- Varies with sodium/water intake
- Regulated by nervous system

Baroreceptors

- Blood pressure sensors via **stretch**
- Signal central nervous system (brain)
- Response via autonomic nervous system
  - Sympathetic and parasympathetic
- Modify:
  - Heart rate/contractility
  - Arterial tone (vasoconstriction)
  - Venous tone (more tone = more preload to ventricle)
  - Renal renin release

Baroreceptors

- Aortic arch and carotid sinus
  - Quick response to changes in blood pressure
  - Rapid response via autonomic nervous system
- Kidneys (renin release)

Baroreceptors

- Aortic arch
  - Senses elevated blood pressure
  - Poor sensing of low blood pressure
- Carotid sinus
  - Most important baroreceptor
  - Modifies signals over wider range of blood pressure
  - Senses low and high blood pressure

Blood Pressure Control

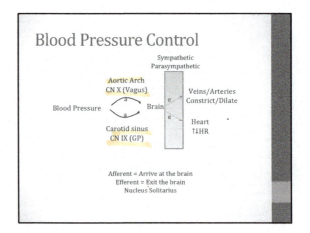

Afferent = Arrive at the brain
Efferent = Exit the brain
Nucleus Solitarius

- Vagus nerve :- Not a good nerve to realize ↑ or ↓ BP.

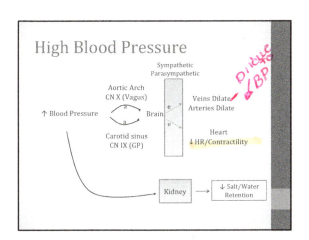

Dilate to ↓ BP

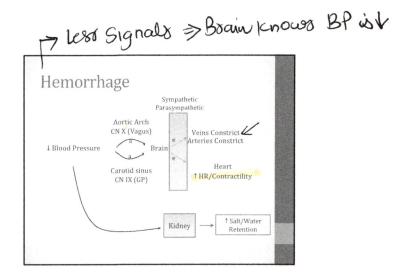

→ Less signals ⇒ Brain knows BP is ↓

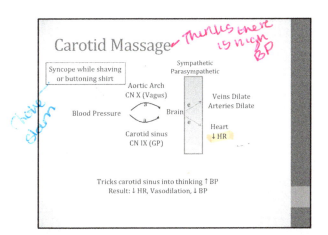

Thinks there is high BP

Pore down

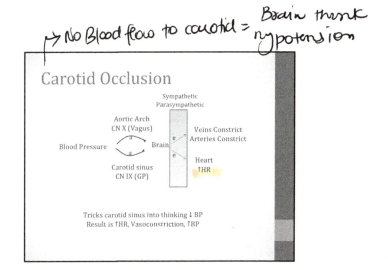

→ No blood flow to carotid = Brain think hypotension

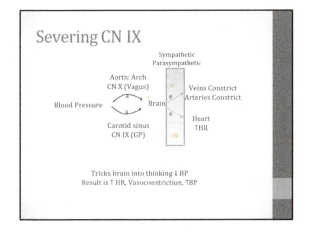

Vagotomy

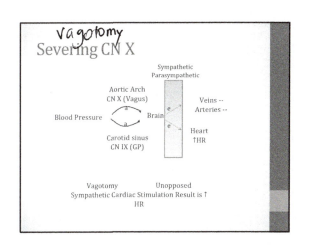

17

Summary of Techniques

hypotension
hypertension

Technique	Interpretation	Result
Carotid Massage	↑BP	↓HR, ↓BP
Carotid Occlusion	↓BP	↑HR, ↑BP
Sever CN IX	↓BP	↑HR, ↑BP
Sever CN X	--	↑HR

Coronary Blood Flow

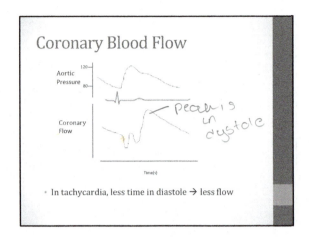

peak is in dystole

- In tachycardia, less time in diastole → less flow

Regional Blood Flow

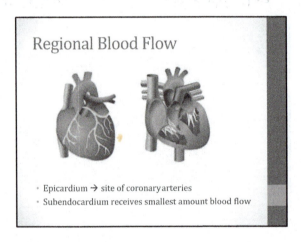

- Epicardium → site of coronary arteries
- Subendocardium receives smallest amount blood flow

Organ Circulation

Organ	Key Features
Lung	100% of Cardiac Output
Liver	Largest Systemic Blood Flow
Kidneys	Highest blood flow by weight
Heart	Largest ΔO2 (80%) ↑ demand vasodilation

Autoregulation

- Some tissue beds maintain **constant blood flow**
- ↑ BP → ↑ flow → vasoconstriction → ↓ flow (normal)
- Use local metabolites to sense blood pressure

Autoregulation

Organ	Key Control Variables
Heart	CO2, Adenosine, NO
Brain	CO2, pH
Kidneys	BP and NaCl feedback
Lungs	Hypoxia → Vasoconstriction
Skeletal Muscle	Lactate, adenosine, K+
Skin	Sympathetic stimulation

Kidney, brain, heart: Excellent autoregulation systems
Skin: Poor autoregulatory capacity

Capillary Fluid Exchange

- Two forces drive fluid into or out of capillaries
- Hydrostatic pressure (P)
  - Molecules against capillaries walls
  - Pushes fluid out
- Oncotic pressure (∏)
  - Solutes (albumin) drawing fluid into capillaries

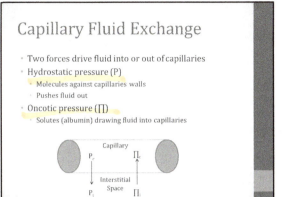

Capillary Fluid Exchange

- Hydrostatic pressure – fluid PUSHING against walls
  - High pressure drives fluid TOWARD low pressure
- Oncotic pressure – solutes PULLING fluid in
  - High pressure draws fluid AWAY from low pressure

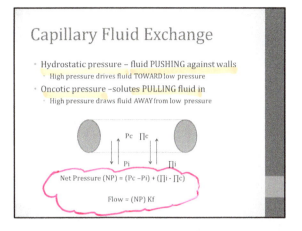

Net Pressure (NP) = (Pc – Pi) + (∏i - ∏c)
Flow = (NP) Kf

Capillary Fluid Exchange

- Hydrostatic pressure – fluid PUSHING against walls
  - High pressure drives fluid TOWARD low pressure
- Oncotic pressure – solutes PULLING fluid in
  - High pressure draws fluid AWAY from low pressure

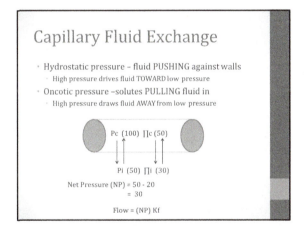

Pc (100) ∏c (50)
Pi (50)   ∏i (30)
Net Pressure (NP) = 50 - 20
                  = 30
Flow = (NP) Kf

Edema

- Excess fluid movement out of capillaries
- Tissue swelling
- Lungs: Pulmonary edema
- Systemic capillaries: Lower extremity edema

James Heilman, MD

Edema

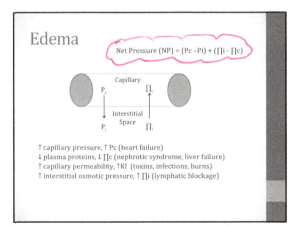

Net Pressure (NP) = (Pc – Pi) + (∏i - ∏c)

↑ capillary pressure, ↑ Pc (heart failure)
↓ plasma proteins, ↓ ∏c (nephrotic syndrome, liver failure)
↑ capillary permeability, ↑Kf (toxins, infections, burns)
↑ interstitial osmotic pressure, ↑ ∏i (lymphatic blockage)

3rd Spacing

- Intracellular fluid – 1st space
  - About 2/3 body fluid
- Extracellular fluid – 2nd space
  - About 1/3 body fluid
- Third spacing - fluid where it should NOT be
  - Pleural effusions
  - Ascites
  - Cerebral edema
  - Low intravascular volume/High total volume
- Occurs post-op, sepsis

Lymphatics usually draws proteins from interstitial, blockage → too much proteins stays in interstitial ⇒ ↑ interstitial osmotic pressure

Pressure Volume Loops

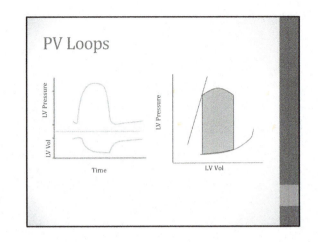

1. End of Systole
2. End of diastole

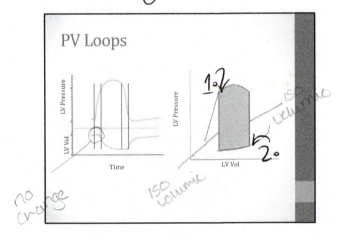

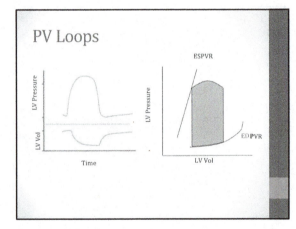

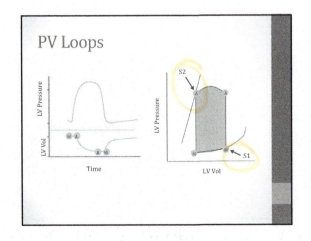

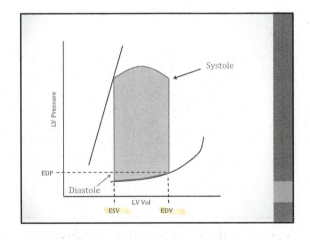

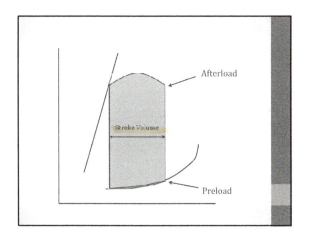

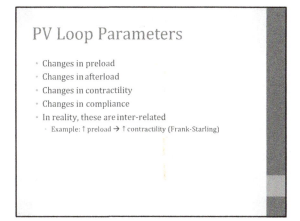

PV Loop Parameters

- Changes in preload
- Changes in afterload
- Changes in contractility
- Changes in compliance
- In reality, these are inter-related
  - Example: ↑ preload → ↑ contractility (Frank-Starling)

Affects EDV

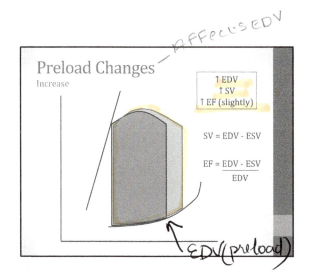

↑ EDV (preload)

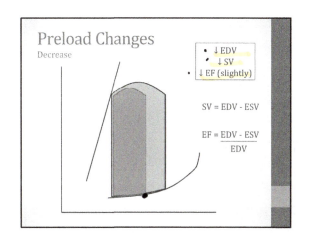

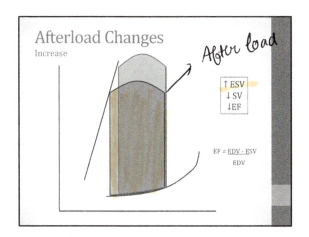

Afterload

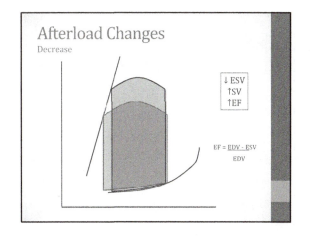

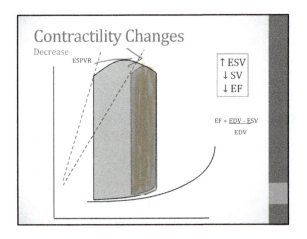
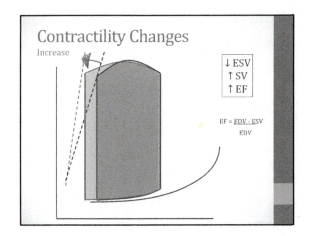
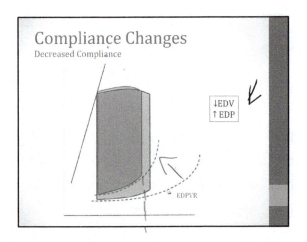
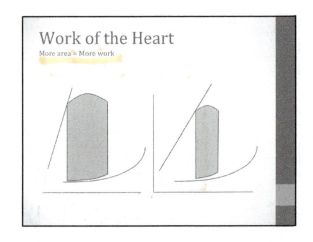

Commonly Tested PV Loops

- Aortic Stenosis
- Mitral Regurgitation
- Aortic Regurgitation
- Mitral Stenosis

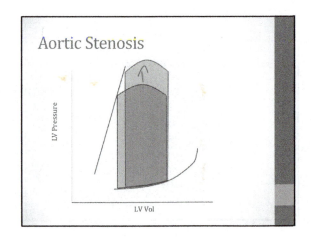

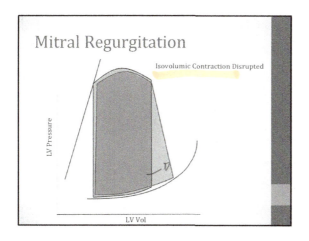
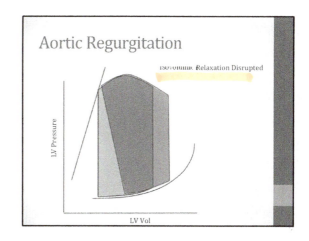
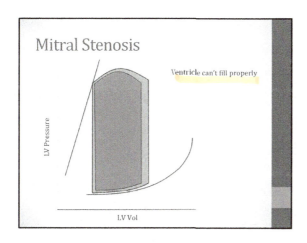

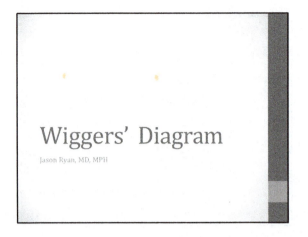

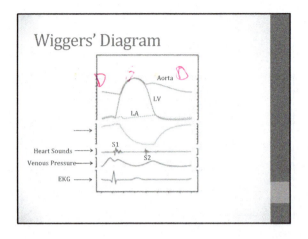

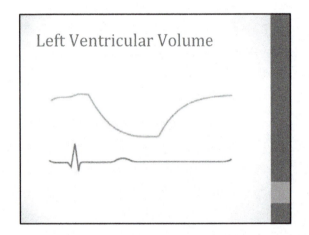

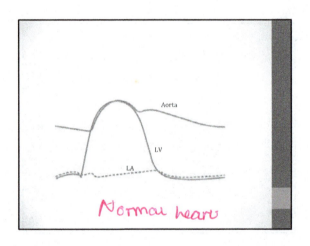

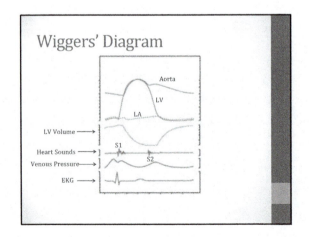

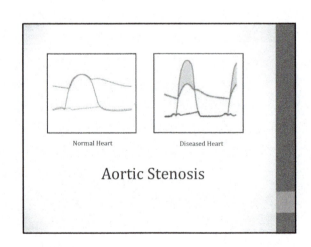

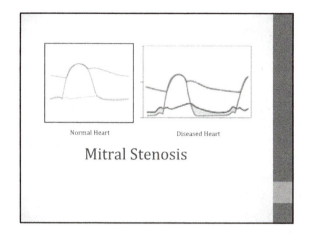

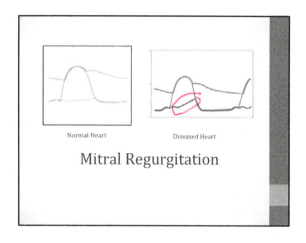

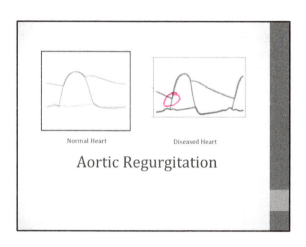

Venous Pressure Tracings

Jason Ryan, MD, MPH

Venous Pressure

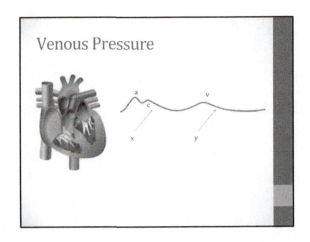

Venous Pressure

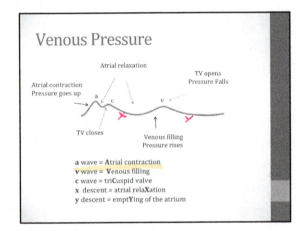

a wave = **A**trial contraction
v wave = **V**enous filling
c wave = tri**C**uspid valve
x descent = atrial rela**X**ation
y descent = empt**Y**ing of the atrium

Venous Pressure
Tricuspid valve

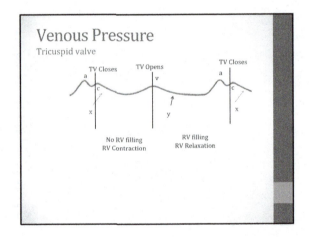

Wiggers' Diagram

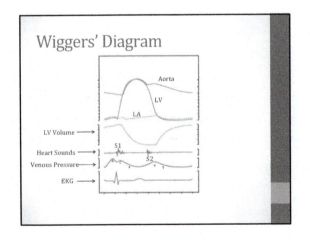

Classic Findings

- Large a wave
- Cannon a wave
- Absent a waves
- Large v waves

Large a wave
Tricuspid stenosis

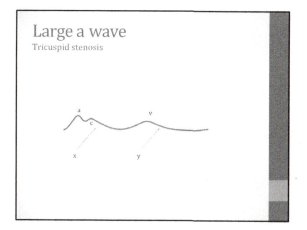

Cannon a wave
AV dissociation

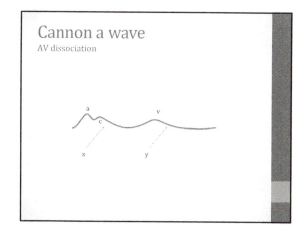

Absent a wave
Atrial fibrillation

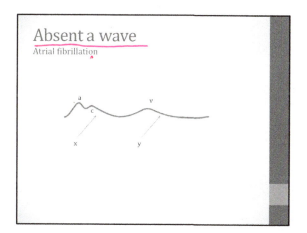

Giant v wave
Tricuspid regurgitation

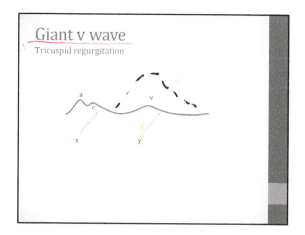

High Yield Findings

- Large a wave (increased atrial contraction pressure)
  - Tricuspid stenosis
  - Right heart failure/Pulmonary hypertension
- Cannon a wave (atria against closed tricuspid valve)
  - Complete heart block
  - PAC/PVC
  - Ventricular tachycardia
- Absent a wave (no organized atrial contraction)
  - Atrial fibrillation
- Giant V waves
  - Tricuspid regurgitation

Left Atrial Pressure

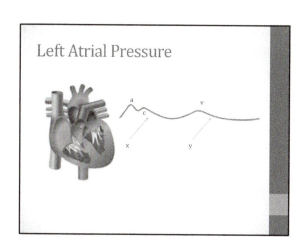

Starling Curves

Jason Ryan, MD, MPH

Frank-Starling Curve

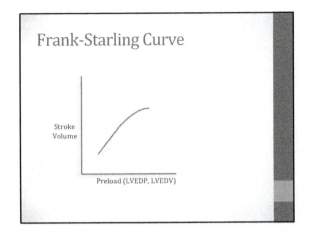

Frank-Starling Curve
Left and Right Shifts

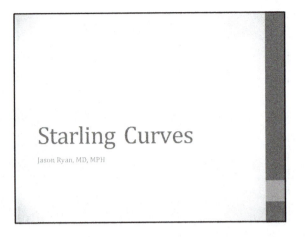

SV = CO
CO = VR

Frank-Starling Curve
Left and Right Shifts

- Contractility
  - Increase: Exercise, inotropes
  - Decrease: Myocardial infarction, heart failure
- Peripheral resistance:
  - Total peripheral resistance (TPR)
  - Systemic vascular resistance (SVR)
  - Increase: Vasopressors
  - Decrease: Vasodilators, sepsis

Venous Return Curve

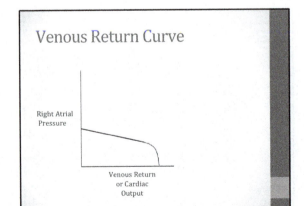

Right Atrial Pressure

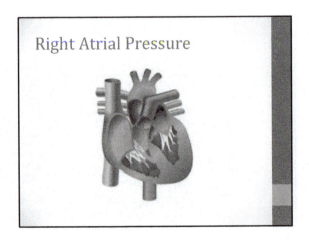

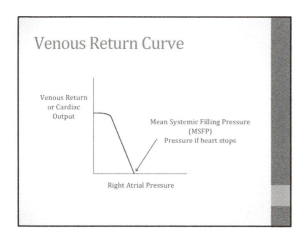
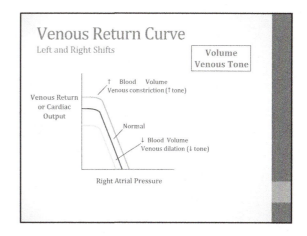
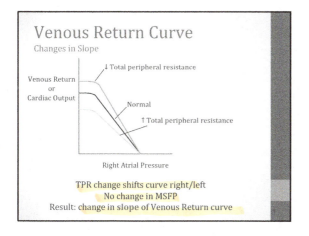
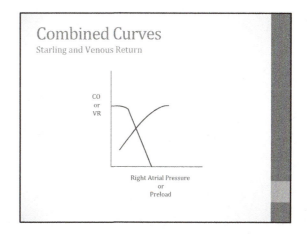
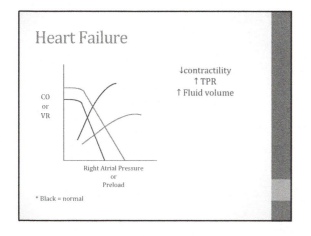
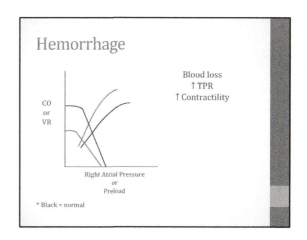

Exercise

- Decreased afterload (TPR)
- Venous contraction
- Increased contractility
- Net result = increased CO

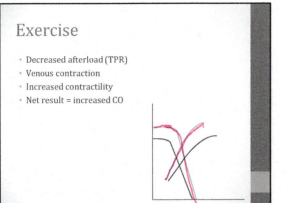

AV Fistulas

- Decreased afterload (TPR)
- Increased contractility
- Venous contraction
- Net result = increased CO

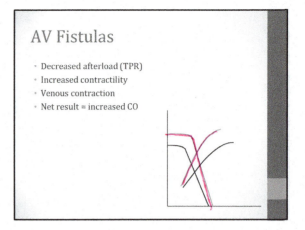

Vasopressors

- Increased afterload (TPR)
- Alters VR and Starling Curves
- Net result = decreased CO

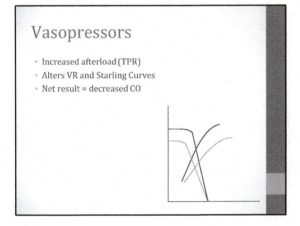

Combined Curves
Starling and Venous Return

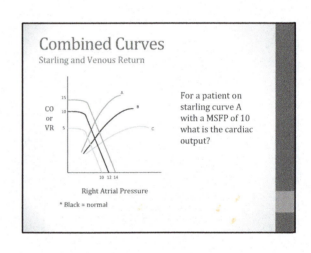

For a patient on starling curve A with a MSFP of 10 what is the cardiac output?

* Black = normal

Atherosclerosis

Jason Ryan, MD, MPH

Vocabulary

- Arteriosclerosis
  - Hardening of arteries
  - Hyaline
  - Hyperplastic
- Atherosclerosis
  - Form of arteriosclerosis
  - Most common type

Atherosclerosis

- Plaque accumulation in arterial walls
- Chronic inflammatory process
- Involves macrophages, T-cells
- Accumulation of lipoproteins especially LDL
- Underlying cause of many diseases
  - Myocardial infarction
  - Stroke
  - Peripheral vascular disease

A. Rad et al./Wikipedia

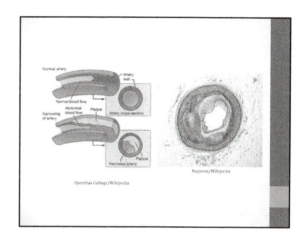

OpenStax College/Wikipedia   Nephron/Wikipedia

Arterial Structure

- Intima
  - Single layer of endothelial cells
  - Basement membrane
- Media
  - Smooth muscle cells
  - Elastin
- Adventicia
  - Connective tissue
  - Vasa vasorum (blood supply to artery wall)
  - Nerve fibers

Bruce Blaus/Wikipedia

Type of Arteries

- Elastic
  - Large amounts of elastin in media layer
  - Expansion in systole, contraction in diastole
  - Aorta, carotid arteries, iliac arteries
- Muscular
  - Layers of smooth muscle cells
  - Vasoconstriction/vasodilation to modify blood flow
  - Arterioles: smallest muscular vessels (most flow resistance)

Atherosclerosis

- **Large elastic arteries**
  - Aorta, carotid arteries, iliac arteries
- **Medium-sized muscular arteries**
  - Coronary, popliteal

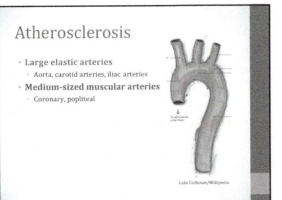

Atherosclerosis
Pathogenesis

- **Endothelial injury or dysfunction**
  - Details incompletely understood
  - Believed to be related to risk factors
  - Cigarette smoke
  - High blood pressure
  - High cholesterol

Atherosclerosis
Pathogenesis

- **Branch points and vessel origins** (ostia)
  - Common sites of plaque
  - Turbulent flow → endothelial stress

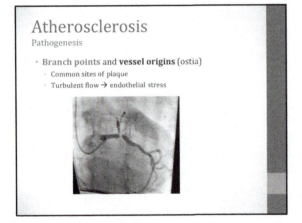

Atherosclerosis
Pathogenesis

- **Lipids**
  - LDL accumulation in intima
  - Oxidized by free radicals
  - Oxidized LDL scavenged by macrophages
  - Cannot be degraded
  - Macrophages become foam cells

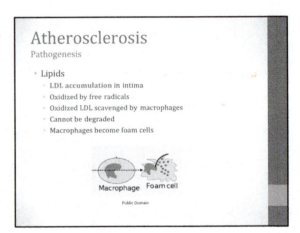

Atherosclerosis
Pathogenesis

- **Chronic inflammation**
  - LDL oxidized from free radicals
  - Damages endothelium, smooth muscle
  - Macrophages release cytokines

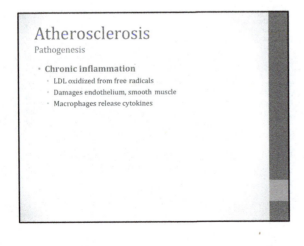

Atherosclerosis
Pathogenesis

- **Smooth muscle cells proliferate in intima**
- Lay down extracellular matrix
- Key growth factor: PDFG
  - Platelet-derived growth factor

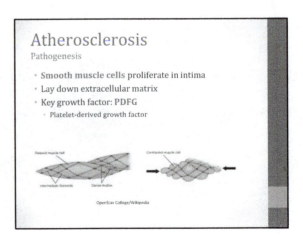

Atheroma Growth

- Fatty streaks
  - Macrophages filled with lipids
  - Form line (steak) along vessel lumen
  - Do not impair blood flow
  - Can be seen in children, adolescents
  - Not all progress

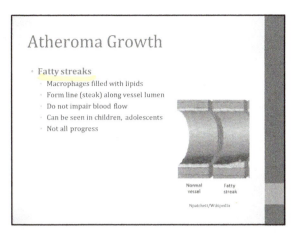

Atheroma Growth

- Atherosclerotic plaques
  - Intima thickens
  - Lipids accumulate
  - Usually patchy along vessel wall
  - Rarely involve entire vessel wall
  - Usually eccentric

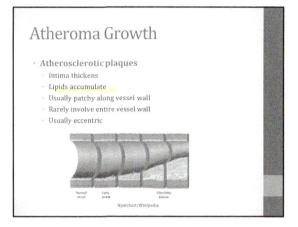

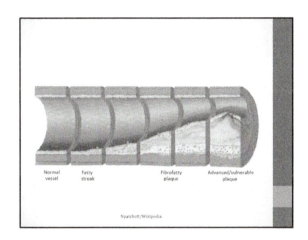

Locations

- Abdominal aorta (large vessel)
- Coronary arteries
- Popliteal arteries
- Internal carotid
- Circle of Willis

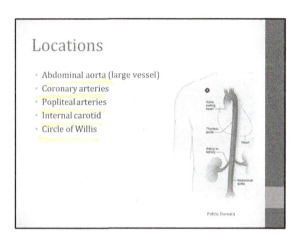

Atherosclerosis Complications

- Ischemia
- Plaque rupture
  - Exposes thrombogenic substances
  - Clot formation
  - May cause acute vessel closure (STEMI)
  - Thrombus may embolize (stroke from carotid plaque)

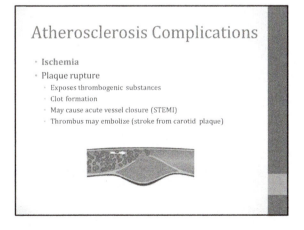

Atherosclerosis Complications

- Hemorrhage into plaque
  - Lesions: proliferating small vessels ("neovascularization")
  - Contained rupture may suddenly expand lesion
- Aneurysm
  - Lesions may damage underlying media
  - Plaque associated with abdominal aortic aneurysms

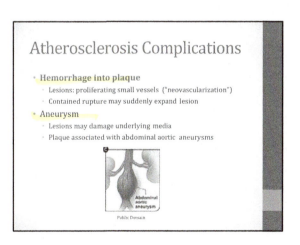

Dystrophic Calcification

- Commonly seen in atheroma
- Result of chronic inflammation
- Basis for "coronary CT scans"

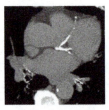

Infarction

- Area of ischemic necrosis
- Two types: white and red
- **White infarcts**
  - Occlusion of arterial supply to a solid organ
  - Common in heart, kidneys, spleen
  - Limited blood seepage from healthy tissue
  - Tissue becomes pale (white)

White Infarct
Renal Infarction

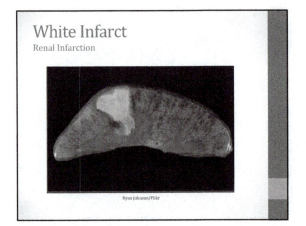

Ryan Johnson/Flikr

Red Infarcts
Hemorrhagic Infarct

- Blood enters ischemic tissue
- Blockage of venous drainage
  - Testicular torsion
- Tissues with dual circulation
  - Blood flow from 2nd supply floods ischemic area
  - Classic location: Lung (diffuse blood supply)
  - Small intestine
- Flow re-established to necrotic area
  - Angioplasty restores flow in coronary artery

Red Infarct
Lung Infarction

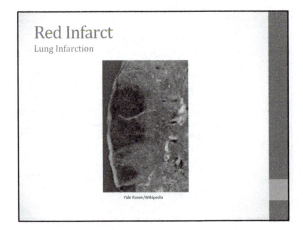

Yale Rosen/Wikipedia

Cardiac Ischemia

Jason Ryan, MD, MPH

Cardiac Ischemia

- Caused by coronary atherosclerosis
- O2 SUPPLY << O2 DEMAND = ISCHEMIA
- Typical symptoms
  - Chest pain (angina)
  - Dyspnea
  - Diaphoresis

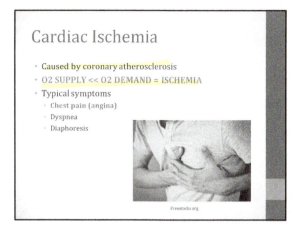

Stable Angina

- Stable atherosclerotic plaque
  - No plaque ulceration
  - No thrombus
- Must occlude ~75% of lumen to cause symptoms

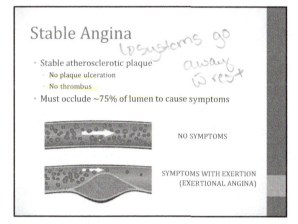

Acute Coronary Syndromes

- Plaque rupture → thrombus formation
- Subtotal occlusion
  - Unstable angina
  - Non-ST elevation myocardial infarction
- Total occlusion (100%)
  - ST-elevation myocardial infarction (STEMI)

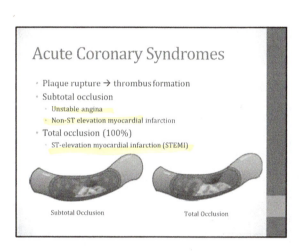

Sudden Death

- Common complication of CAD
- Plaque rupture → arrhythmias
- CAD is most common cause of sudden death adults
  - Younger patients: Hypertrophic cardiomyopathy (HCM)

Risk Factors

- Major risk is prior coronary disease
- Coronary risk equivalents
  - Diabetes
  - Peripheral artery disease
  - Chronic kidney disease

Risk Factors

- Hypertension
- Hyperlipidemia
- Family History (1° relative, M<50, F<60)
- Smoking
- Obesity, sedentary lifestyle

Extent of Ischemia

- Transmural ischemia
  - Occurs with complete 100% flow obstruction (STEMI)
- Subendocardial ischemia
  - Occurs with flow obstruction but some distal blood flow
  - Stable angina, unstable angina, NSTEMI

Subendocardial Ischemia   Transmural Ischemia

Subendocardial Ischemia

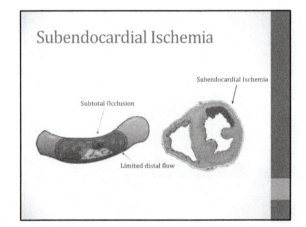

Transmural Ischemia

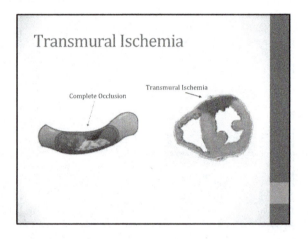

Ischemic EKG changes
ST depressions

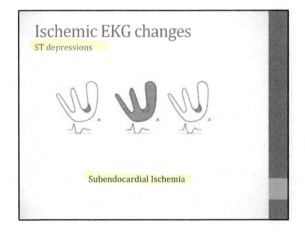

Subendocardial Ischemia

Ischemic EKG changes
T wave inversions

- Many causes other than CAD
- Raised ICP
  - Cerebral T waves
- Resolving pericarditis
- Bundle branch blocks
- Ventricular hypertrophy

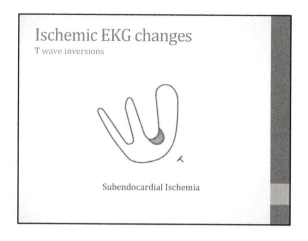

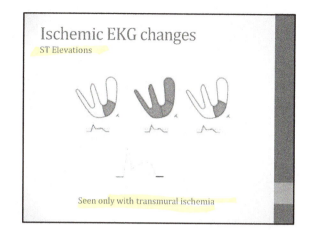

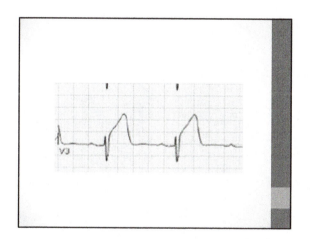

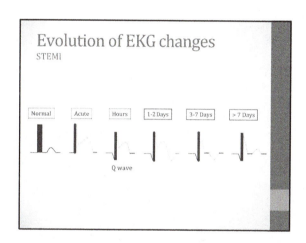

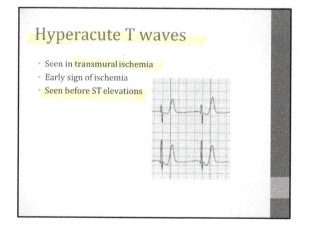

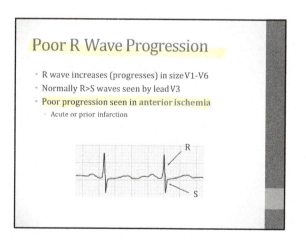

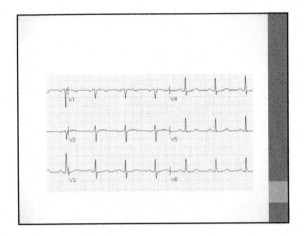

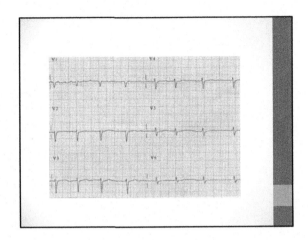

Terminology

- Revascularization — Restore Blood flow
- Angioplasty
- Coronary stenting
- Coronary bypass surgery

Revascularization

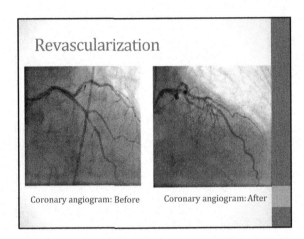

Coronary angiogram: Before   Coronary angiogram: After

Coronary Stents

- Angioplasty: Reshape vessel
- Balloon angioplasty: Balloon inflation to open vessel
- Percutaneous Coronary Intervention (PCI)
- Stent placement
- About 600,000 stents/year implanted US

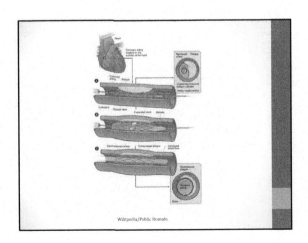

Wikipedia/Public Domain

CABG
Coronary Artery Bypass Surgery

- "Bypass Surgery"
- Left Internal Mammary Artery (LIMA) Graft
- Saphenous (leg) Vein Grafts
- Radial (arm) Artery Grafts

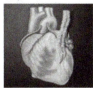

Patrick J. Lynch/Wikipedia

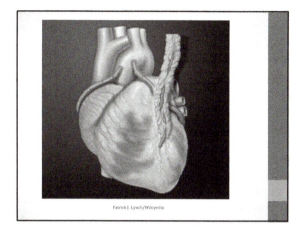

Patrick J. Lynch/Wikipedia

Revascularization
Major Indications

- Angina
- Myocardial infarction
- Systolic dysfunction
  - Hibernating myocardium

Ischemic Pathologic Changes
Myocardium

- Zero to 4 hrs
  - No changes!
- 4 – 12 hrs
  - Gross: Mottled
  - Micro: Necrosis, edema, hemorrhage
- 12-24 hrs — yellow
  - Gross: Hyperemia
  - Micro: Surrounding tissue inflammation
- 5 – 10 days
  - Gross: Central yellowing
  - Micro: Granulation tissue
- 7 weeks
  - Gross: Gray-white scar
  - Micro: Scar

Complications of Ischemia

- First 4 days
  - Arrhythmia
- 5 – 10 days
  - Free wall rupture
  - Tamponade
  - Papillary muscle rupture
  - VSD (septal rupture)
- Weeks later
  - Dressler's syndrome
  - Aneurysm
  - LV Thrombus/CVA

Cause of Death — Arrhythmia
0 – 4 days after MI

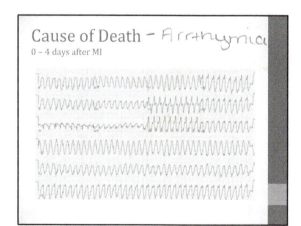

Cause of Death
5-10 days after MI

- **Free wall rupture**
  - Usually fatal – sudden death
  - May lead to tamponade
- **Papillary muscle rupture**
  - Acute mitral regurgitation (holosystolic murmur)
  - Heart failure, respiratory distress
  - More common inferior MIs
- **Septal rupture – VSD**
  - Loud, holosystolic murmur (thrill)
  - Hypotension, right heart failure (↑ JVP, edema)

Ventricular Aneurysm
Weeks after MI

- **More common anterior infarction**
- Risk of thrombus → stroke, peripheral embolism

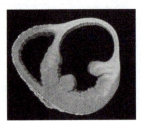

Patrick J. Lynch, medical illustrator/Wikipedia

Ventricular Pseudoaneurysm

- **Rupture contained by pericardium/scar tissue**
- Not a true aneurysm
  - No endocardium or myocardium
- May rupture
- Presents as chest pain or dyspnea
- Often seen in the **inferior wall**
- Occurs earlier (<2 weeks) than true aneurysm

Dressler's Syndrome
Weeks to months after MI

- Form of pericarditis
  - Chest pain
  - Friction rub
- Immune-mediated (details not known)
- Treatment: NSAIDs or steroids

Fibrinous Pericarditis

- Occurs *days* after MI
  - Sometimes called "post-MI" pericarditis
  - Not autoimmune
  - Extension of myocardial inflammation
- **Dressler's occurs *weeks* after MI**
  - Sometimes called "post cardiac injury" pericarditis
- Rarely life-threatening

Secondary Prevention

- Any CAD → ↑ risk of recurrent events
  - STEMI, NSTEMI, stable angina
- Preventative therapy used to lower risk
- Even in asymptomatic patients

Secondary Prevention

- Several proven therapies for risk reduction
- Aspirin
- Statins
  - Atorvastatin, Rosuvastatin
- **Beta blockers**
  - Used in patients with prior infarction (STEMI/NSTEMI)

Stent Complications
Restenosis

- Slow, steady growth of scar tissue over stent
- "Neo-intimal hyperplasia"
- Re-occlusion of vessel
- Rarely life-threatening
- Slow, steady return of angina
- Most stents coated "drug eluting stents"
  - Metal stent covered with polymer
  - Polymer impregnated with drug to prevent tissue growth
  - Sirolimus

Stent Complications
Thrombosis

- Acute closure of stent
- Same as STEMI: life-threatening event
- Dual anti-platelet therapy for prevention
- Associated with **missed medication doses**

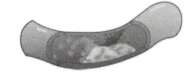

Stent Thrombosis Prevention

- "Dual antiplatelet therapy"
- Typically one year of:
  - Aspirin
  - Clopidogrel, Prasugrel or Ticagrelor
- After one year, stent metal no longer exposed to blood
  - "Endothelialization"
  - Risk of thrombosis is lower (but not zero)
  - Most patients take aspirin only

ST-Elevation Myocardial Infarction (STEMI)

Jason Ryan, MD, MPH

STEMI

- Atherosclerotic plaque rupture
- Thrombus formation
- Ischemic chest pain
- ST-elevations on ECG

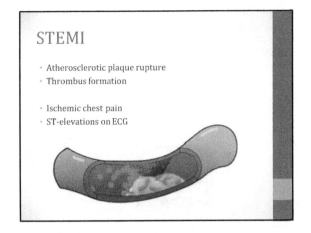

STEMI

- Transmural ischemia

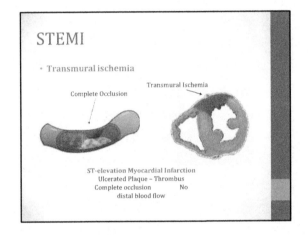

ST-elevation Myocardial Infarction
Ulcerated Plaque – Thrombus
Complete occlusion   No distal blood flow

STEMI

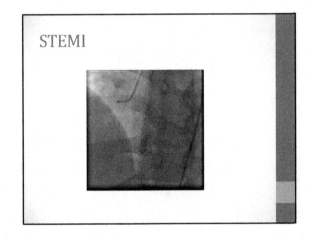

STEMI

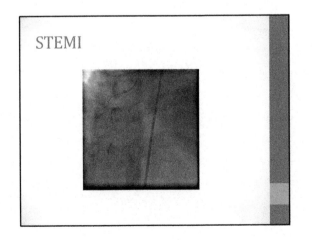

Leads go together
ST Elevations - Anterior

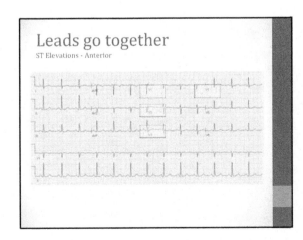

Leads go together
ST Elevations - Anterior

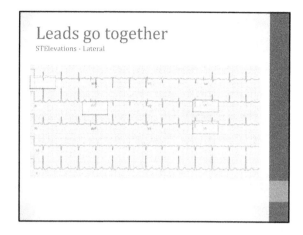

Leads go together
ST Elevations - Lateral

Leads go together
ST Elevations - Lateral

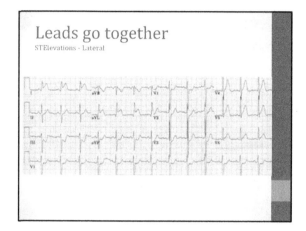

Leads go together
ST Elevations - Inferior

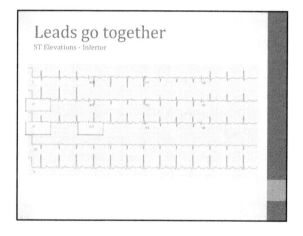

Leads go together
ST Elevations - Inferior

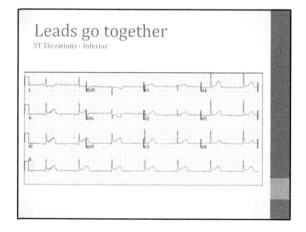

Coronary Artery Territories

- Left anterior descending artery
  - Anterior → V1-V4
- Left circumflex artery
  - Lateral → I, L, V5, V6
- Posterior descending artery
  - Inferior → II, III, F
  - Branch of right coronary artery 90%
  - LCX 10%

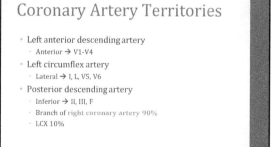

Special Complications
Inferior MI

- Right ventricular infarction
  - Loss of right ventricular contractility
  - Elevated jugular venous pressure
  - Decreased preload to left ventricle → hypotension
  - Diagnosis: Right sided chest leads

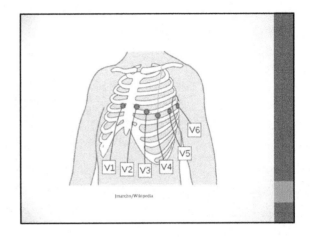

Jmarchn/Wikipedia

Special Complications
Inferior MI

- Sinus bradycardia and heart block
  - Vagal stimulation from inferior wall ischemia

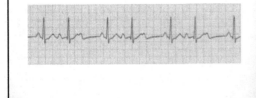

Left Main Occlusion

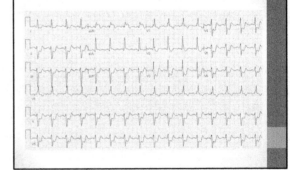

Posterior Myocardial Infarction

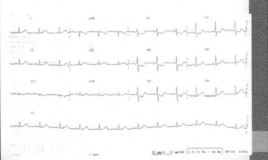

STEMI
Special Subtypes

- Left main
  - ST-elevation aVR
  - Diffuse ST depressions
- Posterior
  - Anterior ST depressions with standard leads
  - ST-elevation in **posterior leads (V7-V9)**

Treatment of STEMI

- "Time is muscle"
- Coronary artery occluded by thrombus
- Longer occlusion → more muscle dies
  - More likely the patient may die
  - More heart failure symptoms
  - More future hospitalization for heart disease
- **Medical emergency**

Treatment of STEMI

- Main objective is to open the artery
  - "Revascularization"
- Option 1: Emergency angioplasty
  - Mechanical opening of artery
  - Should be done <90min
- Option 2: Thrombolysis
  - Lysis of thrombus with drug
  - Should be done <30min
- "Door to balloon" or "door to needle"

Treatment of STEMI

- Time matters
  - Medical therapy is supportive
  - Given while working to open artery
- Remember: this is a <u>thrombotic</u> problem
  - Aspirin to inhibit platelet aggregation
  - Heparin to inhibit clot formation
- This is also an <u>ischemic</u> problem
  - Beta blockers to reduce O2 demand
  - Nitrates to reduce O2 demand

Cautions

- Beta blockers
  - Inferior MI stimulates vagal nerve
  - Bradycardia and AV block can develop
- Nitrates
  - Occlusion of RCA can cause RV infarct
  - RV infarction → ↓ preload
  - Nitrates ↓ preload → hypotension

Other STEMI Treatments

- Clopidogrel
  - ADP receptor blocker
  - Inhibits platelets
- Eptifibatide
  - IIB/IIIA receptor blocker
  - Inhibits platelets
- Bivalirudin
  - Direct thrombin inhibitor
  - Inhibits clot formation

Typical STEMI Course

- Arrival in ER with chest pain 5:42pm
- EKG done 5:50pm
  - STEMI identified
- Cardiac cath lab activated for emergent angioplasty
- Meds given in ER
  - Aspirin
  - Metoprolol
  - Nitro drip
  - Heparin bolus
  - Transport to cath lab 6:15pm
- Artery opened with balloon 6:42pm
  - DTB time 60 minutes (ideal <90min)

Typical STEMI Course

- Arrival in ER with chest pain 5:42pm
- EKG done 5:54pm
  - STEMI identified
- Meds given in ER
  - Aspirin
  - Metoprolol
  - Nitro drip
  - Heparin bolus
- tPA given based on weight 6:07pm
  - IV push
  - Door to needle time 25min (ideal <30)

NSTEMI and Unstable Angina

Jason Ryan, MD, MPH

NSTEMI
Non-ST-Elevation Myocardial Infarction

- Atherosclerotic plaque rupture
- Thrombus formation
- Subtotal (<100%) vessel occlusion
- Ischemic chest pain

Subendocardial Ischemia

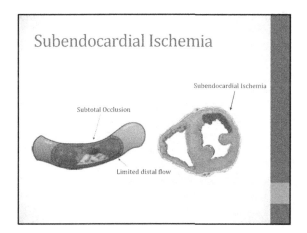

NSTEMI
ECG Changes

- ST depressions
- T-wave inversions

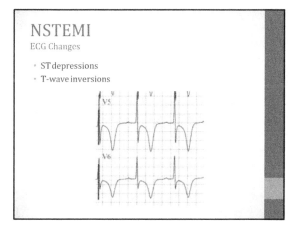

Cardiac Biomarkers

- Biomarkers spill into blood with cardiac injury
- Most common marker used: **Troponin I or T**
  - Increase 2-4 hours after MI
  - Stay elevated for weeks
- **CK-MB also used**
  - Increase 4-6 hours after MI
  - Normalize within 2-3 days

Cardiac Biomarkers

- Several types of CK
  - MM – Skeletal muscle
  - MB – Cardiac
  - BB – Brain
- Most tissues have some of all three
- Ratio of MB to total CK can be used in ischemia
  - Helpful when total CK also up due to muscle damage

Cardiac Biomarkers

- Some AST found in cardiac cells
  - Abdominal pain with isolated ↑ AST could be MI

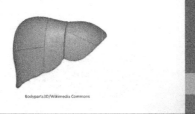

Bodyparts3D/Wikimedia Commons

Treatment of NSTEMI

- Thrombotic and ischemic syndrome (like STEMI)
- Unlike STEMI: No "ticking clock"
  - Subtotal occlusion
  - Some blood flow to distal myocardium
  - No emergency angioplasty
  - No benefit to thrombolysis
- Aspirin
- Beta blocker
- Heparin
- Angioplasty (non-emergent)

Typical NSTEMI Course

- Presents to ER with chest pain
- Biomarkers elevated
- Medical Therapy
  - Aspirin
  - Metoprolol
  - Heparin drip
- Admitted to cardiac floor
- Hospital day 2 → angiography
- 90% blockage of LAD → Stent

Unstable Angina

- Atherosclerotic plaque rupture
- Thrombus formation
- Subtotal (<100%) vessel occlusion
- Ischemic chest pain
- **Normal biomarkers**

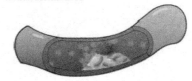

Unstable Angina

- Diagnosis largely based on **patient history**
  - Chest pain increasing in frequency/intensity
  - Chest pain at rest
- ECG may show ST depressions or T wave inversions
- Treatment is same as for NSTEMI
- Condition often called "UA/NSTEMI"

Stable Angina

Jason Ryan, MD, MPH

Stable Angina

- Ischemic chest pain with exertion
- Relieved by rest
- Stable pattern over time
- Stable coronary atherosclerotic plaque
- No plaque rupture/thrombus

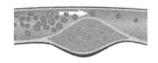

Stable Angina

- Symptoms generally absent until ~75% occlusion
- Distal arteriolar dilation → normal flow if <75%

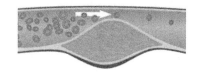

Stable Angina

- Diagnosis: cardiac stress test
- Increases demand for O2

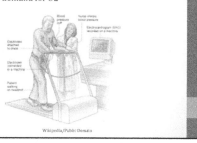

Wikipedia/Public Domain

Stable Angina

- NOT a thrombotic problem
- No role for heparin or antithrombotic drugs
- In US usually treated with revascularization
  - Most common indication PCI, CABG is stable angina
  - Recent clinical trials suggest medical therapy may work just as well as PCI/CABG in some patients

Stable Angina: Typical Case

- 65-year old man with chest pain while walking
- Relieved with rest
- Presents to ED
  - EKG normal
  - Biomarkers normal
- Stress test
  - Walks on treadmill → chest pain, EKG changes
- Cardiac catheterization performed
- 90% LAD artery blockage
- Stent placed → angina resolved

Medical Therapy for Ischemia

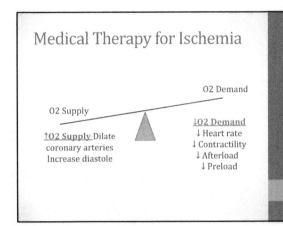

↑O2 Supply Dilate coronary arteries
Increase diastole

↓O2 Demand
↓ Heart rate
↓ Contractility
↓ Afterload
↓ Preload

Nitrates

- Converted to nitric oxide → vasodilation
- Predominant mechanism is **venous dilation**
  - Bigger veins hold more blood
  - Takes blood away from left ventricle
  - Lowers preload (LVEDV)
- Also arterial vasodilation (art << veins)
  - Increase coronary perfusion
  - Some peripheral vasodilation

Nitroglycerine

Nitrates

- ↓ preload → ↓ cardiac output
- **Sympathetic nervous system activation**
- Increased heart rate/contractility
  - Increases O2 demand
  - Opposite of what we want to do for angina

Nitrates

- Rare patients with complex CAD → angina
- In most patients, preload reducing effects dominate
  - Nitrates alone often improve angina
- **Co-administer beta-blocker or Ca channel blocker**
  - Blunts "reflex" effect

Nitrates
Forms

- Nitroglycerin Tablets/Spray
  - Rapid action ~5 minutes
  - Take during angina attack, before exercise
- Isosorbide Dinitrate
  - Effects last ~6hrs
- Isosorbide Mononitrate
  - Once daily drug
- Topical Nitroglycerin
  - Topical cream, patches

Nitrates
Adverse Effects

- Headache (meningeal vasodilation)
- Flushing
- Hypotension
- Angina
  - Reflex sympathetic activation

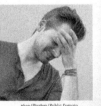

phee/Pixabay/Public Domain

Nitrate Tolerance

- Drug stops working after frequent use
- Avoid continuous us for more than 24 hours
- Does not occur with daily isosorbide mononitrate

Nitrate Withdrawal

- Nitrate withdrawal (rebound) after discontinuation
- Occurs when using large doses of long-acting nitrates
- Angina frequency will increase

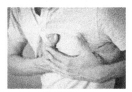

Monday Disease

- Workers in nitroglycerin manufacturing facilities
- Regular exposure to NTG in the workplace
- Leads to the development of tolerance
- Over the weekend workers lose the tolerance
- "Monday morning headache" phenomenon
  - Re-exposed on Monday
  - Prominent vasodilation
  - Tachycardia, dizziness, and a headache

Beta Blockers

- Slow heart rate and decrease contractility
- Increase preload (LVEDV)
  - Slower heart rate = more filling time
  - Increase O2 demand
  - Blunts some beneficial effect
- Reduced blood pressure (↓ afterload)
- **Net effect = less O2 demand**

Beta Blockers

- For angina, generally use cardioselective (β1) drugs
  - Metoprolol, atenolol
- Some beta blockers are partial agonists
  - Pindolol, Acebutolol
  - Don't use in angina

Calcium Channel Blockers

- Three major classes of calcium antagonists
  - dihydropyridines (nifedipine)
  - phenylalkylamines (verapamil)
  - benzothiazepines (diltiazem)
- Vasodilators and negative inotropes

Calcium Channel Blockers

- **Nifedipine: vasodilator**
  - Lower blood pressure
  - Reduce afterload
  - Dilate coronary arteries
  - May cause reflex tachycardia
- **Verapamil/diltiazem: negative inotropes**
  - Similar to beta blockers
  - Reduced heart rate/contractility
  - Can precipitate acute heart failure if LVEF very low

Antianginal Therapy
Nitrates/Beta Blockers

	Nitrates	Beta blockers	Nitrates + Beta blockers
Supply			
Coronary vasodilation	Increase	--	Increase
Duration diastole	↓ reflex	Increase	--
Demand			
Preload	Decrease	Increase	Decrease
Afterload	Decrease	Decrease	Decrease
Contractility	↑ reflex	Decrease	--/↓
Heart Rate	↑ reflex	Decrease	--/↓

Antianginal Therapy
Calcium Channel Blockers

	Verapamil	Diltiazem	Nifedipine
Supply			
Coronary vasodilation	--	--	Increase
Duration diastole	Increase	Increase	↓ reflex
Demand			
Preload	Increase	Increase	--
Afterload	Decrease	Decrease	Decrease
Contractility	Decrease	Decrease	↑ reflex
Heart Rate	Decrease	Decrease	↑ reflex

Ranolazine

- Inhibits **late sodium current**
- Reduces calcium overload → high wall tension
- Reduces wall tension and O2 demand

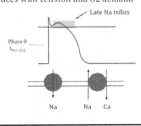

Ranolazine

- Constipation, dizziness, headache
- QT prolongation (blockade of K channels)

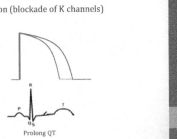

Prolong QT

Variant (Prinzmetal) Angina

- Ischemia from **vasospasm**
  - Not caused by atherosclerotic narrowing
  - Often artery is "clean" with no stenosis
  - May also occur near sites of mild atherosclerosis
- Spontaneous episodes of angina
- Transient myocardial ischemia
- **ST-segment elevation on ECG**

Variant (Prinzmetal) Angina

- Episodes usually **at rest**
- Midnight to early morning
- Sometimes symptoms improve with exertion
- Associated with smoking

Variant (Prinzmetal) Angina
Diagnosis

- Usually based on history
- Intracoronary **ergonovine**
  - Acts on smooth muscle serotonergic (5-HT2) receptors
  - Can be administered during angiography
  - Vasospasm visualized on angiogram
- Intracoronary **acetylcholine**
  - Acts on endothelial muscarinic receptors
  - Healthy endothelium → vasodilation via nitric oxide
  - Endothelial dysfunction → vasoconstriction
  - Vasospasm visualized on angiogram

Variant (Prinzmetal) Angina
Treatment

- Quit smoking
- Calcium channel blockers, nitrates
  - Vasodilators
  - Dilate coronary arteries, oppose spasm
- **Avoid propranolol**
  - Non selective blocker
  - Can cause unopposed alpha stimulation
  - Symptoms may worsen

Pixabay/Public Domain

Coronary Steal

- Mechanism of angina
- Induced by drugs
- Blood flow increased to healthy vessels
- Blood flow decreased in stenotic vessels
- Blood "stolen" from diseased coronary vessels

Coronary Steal

- Stenotic vessels
  - Significant (>75%) narrowing
  - Arterioles maximally dilated to maintain flow
- Normal vessels
  - No or minimal narrowing
  - **Arterioles NOT maximally dilated**

Coronary Steal

- **Vasodilator administered**
- Stenotic vessels → no response
  - Arterioles already maximally dilated
- Normal vessels → vasodilation
- Flow increases to normal vessels
- Flow decreases to abnormal vessels
- Results: ischemia due to coronary steal

Coronary Steal

- Rarely seen with nitrates, nifedipine
- Key principle for **chemical stress tests**
  - Adenosine, persantine, regadenoson
  - Potent, short-acting vasodilators
  - Brief ↓ in blood flow to stenotic vessels → ischemia
  - Nuclear tracers can detect ↓ blood flow

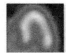
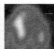

EKG Basics

Jason Ryan, MD, MPH

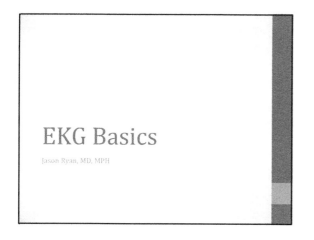
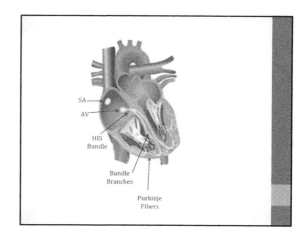
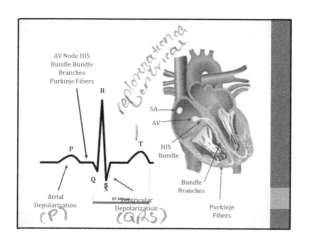
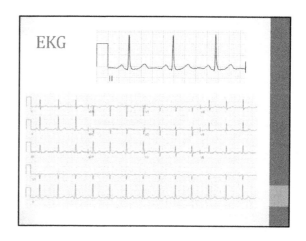

EKG Electrical Activity

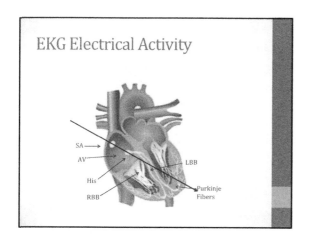

EKG Electrical Activity

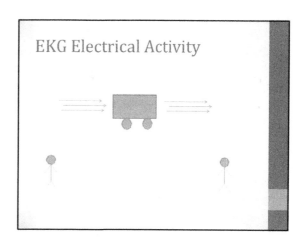

EKG Electrical Activity

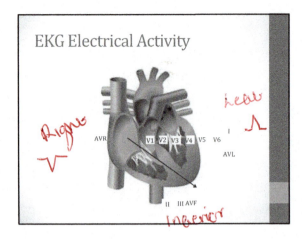

Handwritten annotations: "Right" (pointing to AVR side), "Left" (pointing to I/AVL side), "Inferior" (pointing to II/III/AVF)

EKG

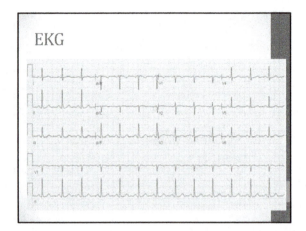

EKGs
Key Principles

- #1: Waves represent repolarization/depolarization
- #2: EKGs have 12 leads
  - Each lead watches the same thing
  - Each lead watches from different vantage point
  - Electrical activity toward lead = upward deflection
  - Electrical activity away from lead = negative deflection

Pacemakers

- SA node is dominant pacemaker of the heart
- Other pacemakers exist but are *slower*
- If SA node fails, others takeover
  - SA node (60-100 bpm)
  - AV node (40-60 bpm)
  - HIS (25-40 bpm)
  - Bundle branches (25-40 bpm)
  - Purkinje fibers (25-40 bpm)

Conduction Velocities

- SLOWEST conduction is through AV node
  - Very important so ventricle has time to fill
- Purkinje fibers → fastest conduction
- Purkinje > Atria > Vent > AV node

Determining Heart Rate

- 3 – 5 big boxes between QRS complex

Handwritten: "# Big Box / 300"

300 150 100 75 60 50

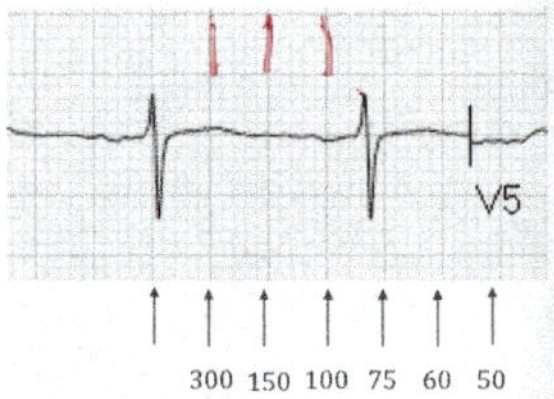

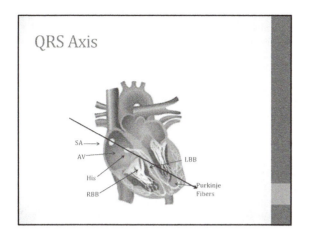
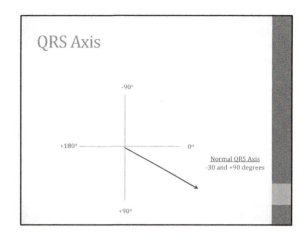
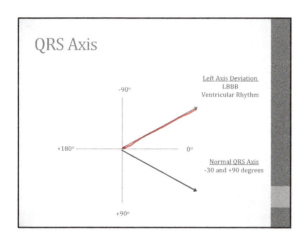
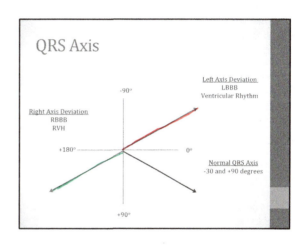
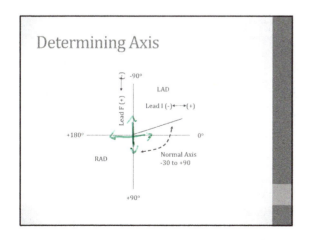
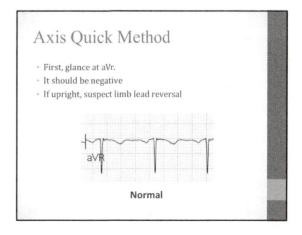

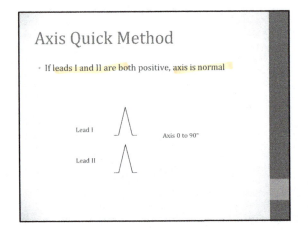
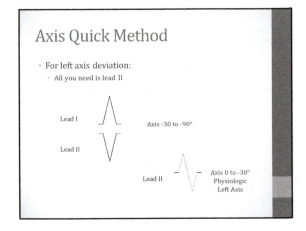
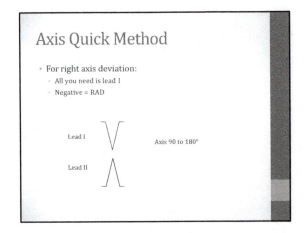
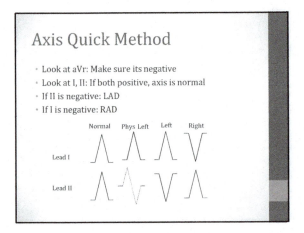
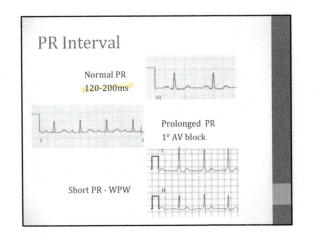
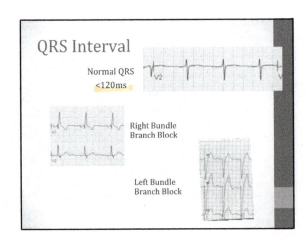

Qt Interval

Normal Qt

Short Qt: Hypercalcemia

Prolonged Qt
Hypocalcemia
Drugs
LQTS

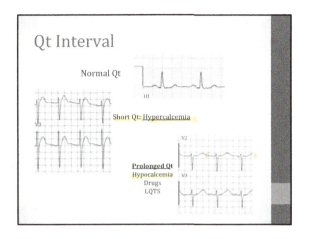

Calcium
Myocyte Action Potential

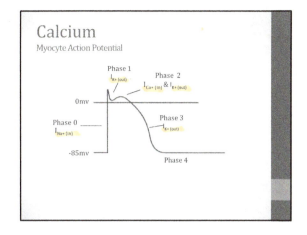

Torsade de Pointes

- Feared outcome of Qt prolongation
- Results in cardiac arrest
- Antiarrhythmic drugs
- Hypokalemia, hypomagnesemia
- Rarely from hypocalcemia

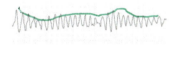

Congenital Long Qt Syndrome

- Rare genetic disorder
  - Abnormal K/Na channels

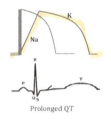

Prolonged QT

Congenital Long Qt Syndrome

- Family history of sudden death (torsades)
- Classic scenario: Young patient recurrent "seizures"
  - EKG shows long Qt interval
- Jervell and Lange-Nielsen Syndrome
  - Norway and Sweden
  - Congenital deafness

Acquired Long Qt Syndrome

- Antiarrhythmic drugs
- Levofloxacin (antibiotic)
- Haldol (antipsychotic)
- Many other drugs
- Congenital LQTS: need to avoid these drugs

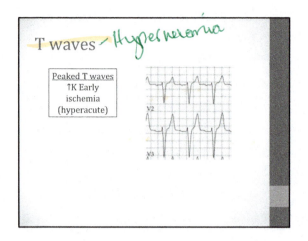
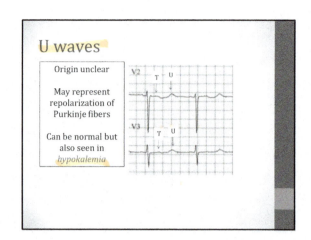

T waves — Hyperkalemia

Peaked T waves
↑K Early ischemia (hyperacute)

U waves

Origin unclear

May represent repolarization of Purkinje fibers

Can be normal but also seen in *hypokalemia*

High Yield EKGs

Jason Ryan, MD, MPH

EKGs You Should Know

1. Sinus rhythm
2. Atrial Fibrillation/Flutter
3. Ischemia: ST elevations, ST depressions
4. Left bundle branch block
5. Right bundle branch block
6. PAC/PVC
7. 1st, 2nd, 3rd degree AV block
8. Ventricular tachycardia
9. Ventricular fibrillation/Torsades

Step 1: Find the p waves

- Are p waves present?

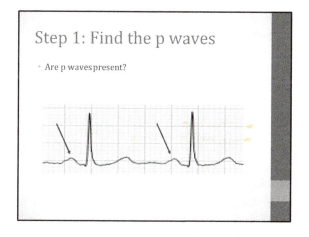

Sinus p waves

- Originate in sinus node
- Upright in leads II, III, F

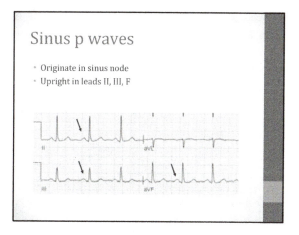

Step 2: Regular or Irregular

- Distance between QRS complexes (R-R intervals)

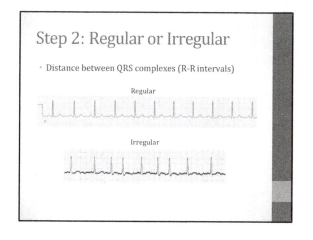

Steps 1 & 2

- P waves present, regular rhythm
  - Sinus rhythm
  - Rare: atrial tachycardia, atrial rhythm
- No p waves, irregular rhythm
  - Atrial fibrillation – irregularly irregular
  - Atrial flutter with variable block

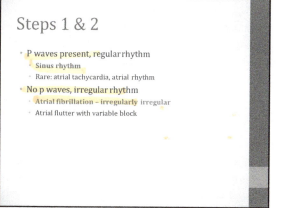

Steps 1 & 2

- P waves present, irregular rhythm
  - Sinus rhythm with PACs
  - Multifocal atrial tachycardia
  - Sinus with AV block
- No p waves, regular rhythm
  - Hidden p waves: retrograde
  - Supraventricular tachycardias (SVTs)
  - Ventricular tachycardia

Step 3: Wide or narrow

- Narrow QRS (<120ms; 3 small boxes)
  - His-Purkinje system works
  - No bundle branch blocks present
- Wide QRS
  - Most likely a bundle branch block
  - Ventricular rhythm (i.e. tachycardia)

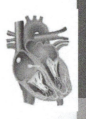

QRS Interval

Normal QRS

Right Bundle Branch Block

Left Bundle Branch Block

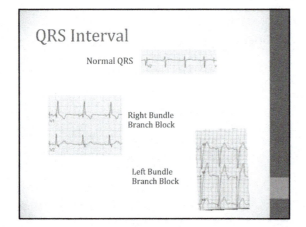

Step 4: Check the intervals

- PR (normal <210ms; ~5 small boxes; ~1 big box)
  - Prolonged in AV block
  - Lengthens with vagal tone, drugs
  - Shortens with sympathetic tone
- QT (normal <1/2 R-R interval)
  - Prolonged with ↓ Ca (tetany; numbness; spasms)
  - Prolonged by antiarrhythmic drugs
  - Shortened with ↑ Ca (confusion, constipation)

Step 5: ST segments

- T wave abnormalities
  - Inverted: ischemia
  - Peaked: Early ischemia, hyperkalemia (↑K)
  - Flat/U waves: Hypokalemia (↓K)
- ST Depression
  - Subendocardial ischemia
- ST Elevation
  - Transmural ischemia

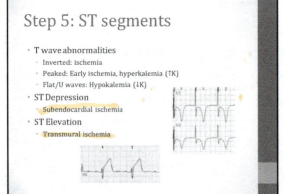

Normal Sinus Rhythm

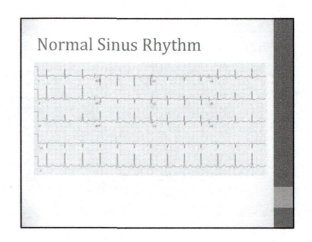

Right Bundle Branch Block

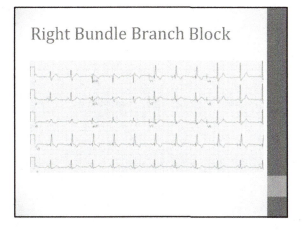

Left Bundle Branch Block

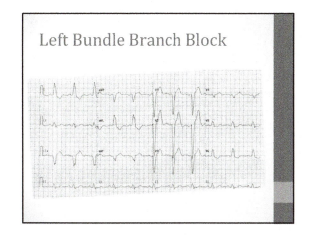

Atrial Fibrillation (No 'P' waves)

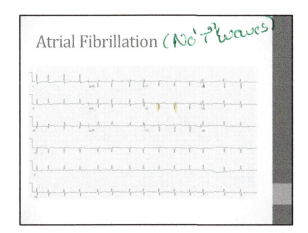

Atrial Flutter

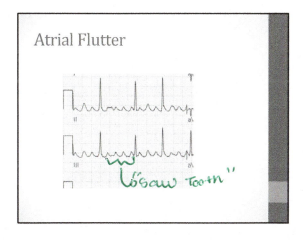

"Saw Tooth"

Ventricular Tachycardia

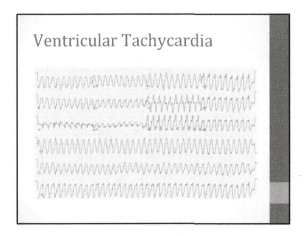

Ventricular Tachycardia

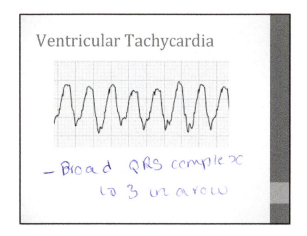

- Broad QRS complex
- 3 in a row

Torsades de pointes

- ↑ risk with **prolonged Qt interval**
  - Antiarrhythmic drugs
  - Congenital long Qt syndrome
  - Antibiotics (erythromycin, quinolones)
- Hypokalemia
- Hypomagnesemia
- Rarely hypocalcemia

Ventric Fibrillation

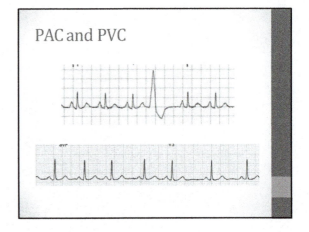

Cardiac Action Potentials

Jason Ryan, MD, MPH

Cardiac Action Potential

- Changes in membrane voltage of cell
- Transmit electrical signals through heart
- Triggers contraction of myocytes

Myocyte Action Potential
Atrial/ventricular myocytes

- Phase 1: $I_{K+ (out)}$
- Phase 2: $I_{Ca2+ (in)}$ & $I_{K+ (out)}$
- Phase 0: $I_{Na+ (in)}$
- Phase 3: $I_{K+ (out)}$
- Phase 4

Phase 4

- Resting potential: about −85mV
- Constant outward leak of K^+
- "Inward rectifier channels"
- Na^+ and Ca^{2+} channels are closed

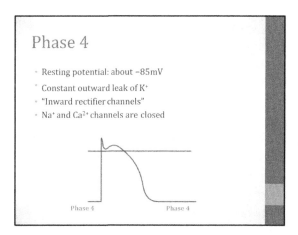

Phase 0

- Nearby myocyte raise membrane potential
- Gap junctions
- Rising potential opens "Fast" Na^+ channels
- Threshold potential reached (about -70mV)
- Large Na^+ current → rapid depolarization
- Membrane potential overshoots (>0mV)
- Fast Na^+ channels close
- **Class I antiarrhythmic drugs**: block Na channels

Phase 1

- Membrane potential is positive
- K^+ channels open
- Outward flow of K^+ returns membrane to ~0 mV

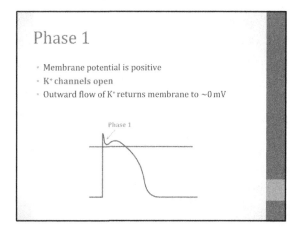

Phase 2

- L-type Ca^{2+} channels open → inward Ca^{2+} current
- Contraction trigger: **excitation-contraction coupling**
- K^+ leaks out (down concentration gradient)
- Delayed rectifier K^+ channels
- **Balanced flow in/out = plateau of membrane charge**
- **Verapamil/Diltiazem** = block L-type Ca channels

Phase 3

- Ca^{2+} channels inactivated
- **Persistent outflow of K^+**
- Resting potential back to −85 mV
- **Class III antiarrhythmic drugs**: block K channels

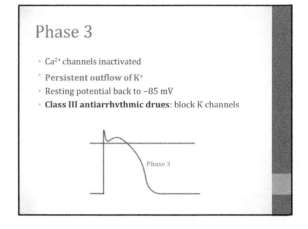

Skeletal Muscle

- No plateau (phase 2)
- No gap junctions
- Each cell has its own NMJ

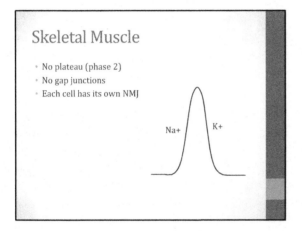

Refractory Period

- Phase 0 until next possible depolarization
- Determines how fast myocyte can conduct
- Many antiarrhythmic drugs prolong refractory period

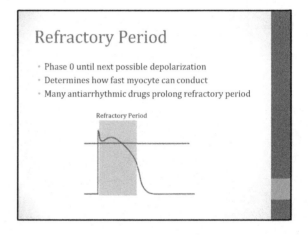

Myocyte Action Potential
Atrial/ventricular myocytes

- Similar AP in HIS, bundle branches, Purkinje fibers

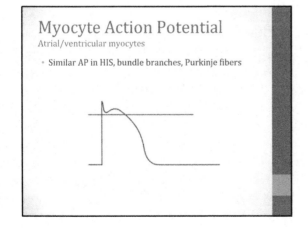

Pacemaker Action Potential
SA node, AV node

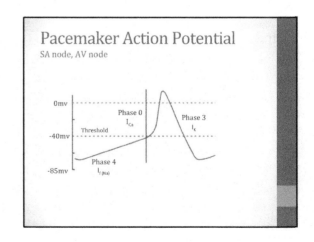

Pacemaker Action Potential
SA node, AV node

- **Funny current** (pacemaker current)
  - Spontaneous flow of Na⁺
- About –40 mV: threshold potential
- L-type Ca^{2+} channels open → depolarize cell
- Delayed rectifier K⁺ channels open
- Return cell to –60 mV

Pacemaker Action Potential
SA node, AV node

- Automaticity
  - Do not require stimulation to initiate action potential
  - Capable of self-initiated depolarization
- No fast Na⁺ channel activity
  - Fewer inward rectifier K⁺ channels
  - Membrane potential never lower than –60 mV
  - Fast Na⁺ channels need –85 mV to function

Pacemaker Action Potential
SA node, AV node

- Any drug that slows this AP may cause two effects:
  - Slower heart rate (sinus node)
  - Slower AV conduction (AV node)

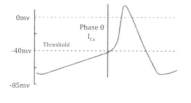

Pacemaker Action Potential
SA node, AV node

- Two key drug classes that affect pacemaker AP
  - **Calcium channel blockers** (Verapamil/Diltiazem)
  - Beta blockers

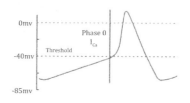

Pacemaker Action Potential
SA node, AV node

- **Verapamil/Diltiazem** = block L-type Ca channels
  - Slow rate of sinus depolarization (slow heart rate)
  - Slow AV node conduction

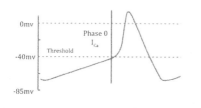

Beta Blockers

- Modify slope of phase 4
- Less slope → longer to reach threshold → ↓HR

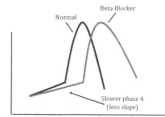

Beta Blockers

- Also prolong repolarization
- Slow AV node conduction

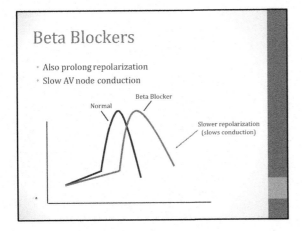

Slope of Phase 4
Sinus Node

- Changes in slope modify heart rate
- Decrease slope (slower rise)
  - Parasympathetic NS, beta blockers, adenosine
- Increased slope (faster rise)
  - Sympathetic NS, sympathomimetic drugs

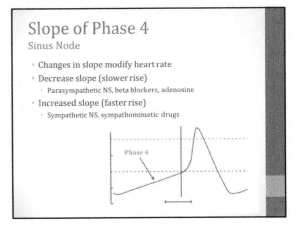

Pacemakers

- Many cardiac cells capable of automaticity
- SA node normally dominates
  - Fastest rise in phase 4
  - Controls other pacemaker cells
- Pacemakers: SA Node > AV Node > Bundle of HIS
  - SA node (60-100 bpm)
  - AV node (40-60 bpm)
  - HIS (25-40 bpm)

AV and Bundle Branch Blocks

Jason Ryan, MD, MPH

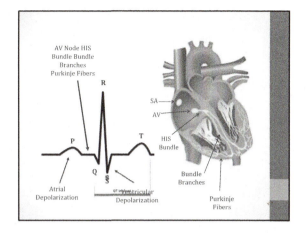

AV Blocks

- Slowed or blocked conduction atria → ventricles
- Can cause <mark>prolonged PR interval</mark> *and fixed*
- Can cause <mark>non-conducted p wave</mark>

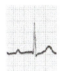

Prolonged PR Interval | Non-conducted P wave

Prolonged → more than 5 boxes

AV Blocks
Symptoms

- Often incidentally noted on EKG
  - Especially milder forms with few/no non-conducted p waves
- Can cause bradycardia
  - Occurs when many or all p waves not conducted
  - Fatigue, dizziness, syncope
  - Symptomatic AV block often treated with a pacemaker

AV Blocks
Anatomy

- Caused by disease in AV conduction system
  - AV node → HIS → Bundle Branches → Purkinje fibers
- Divided into two causes
  - AV node disease
  - HIS-Purkinje disease

AV Blocks
Anatomy

- AV node disease
  - Usually less dangerous
  - Conduction improves with exertion (sympathetic activity)
- HIS-Purkinje disease
  - More dangerous
  - Usually does not improve with exertion
  - Often progresses to complete heart block
  - Often requires a pacemaker

Normal / 1010 Block / WPR

AV Blocks
Four Types

- Type 1
  - Prolongation of PR interval only
  - All p waves conducted
- Type II
  - Some p waves conducted
  - Some p waves NOT conducted
  - Two sub-types: Mobitz I and Mobitz II
- Type III
  - No impulse conduction from atria to ventricles

1st degree AV Block

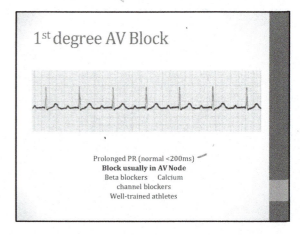

Prolonged PR (normal <200ms)
Block usually in AV Node
Beta blockers Calcium channel blockers
Well-trained athletes

2nd degree AVB
Mobitz I/Wenckebach

Signal never Reached ventricle
NO QRS
Drop Beat

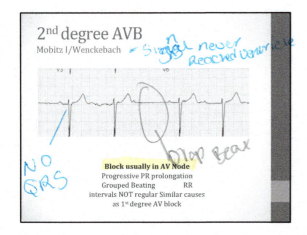

Block usually in AV Node
Progressive PR prolongation
Grouped Beating RR intervals NOT regular Similar causes as 1st degree AV block

2nd degree AVB
Mobitz I/Wenckebach

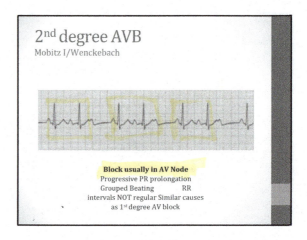

Block usually in AV Node
Progressive PR prolongation
Grouped Beating RR intervals NOT regular Similar causes as 1st degree AV block

2nd degree AVB — *more serious*
Mobitz II

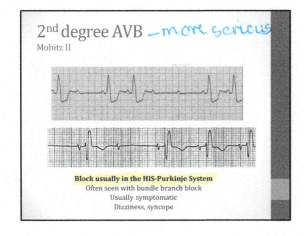

Block usually in the HIS-Purkinje System
Often seen with bundle branch block
Usually symptomatic
Dizziness, syncope

3rd degree AVB

- P & QRS Rate are different
- Lyme disease, Need pacemaker

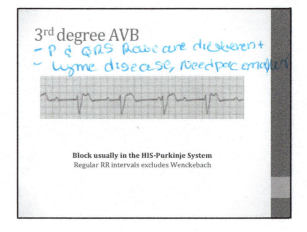

Block usually in the HIS-Purkinje System
Regular RR intervals excludes Wenckebach

3rd degree AVB — cannon waves

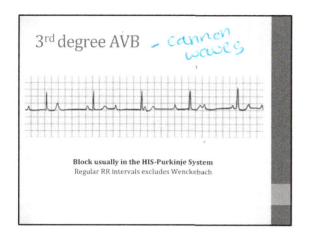

Block usually in the HIS-Purkinje System
Regular RR intervals excludes Wenckebach

Lyme Disease

- Spirochete infection with Borrelia burgdorferi
- Stage 2: Lyme carditis
- Varying degrees of AV block
  - 1st, 2nd, 3rd
- AV block improves with antibiotics

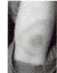

Image courtesy of Wikipedia/Public Domain

Vocabulary

- **Complete heart block**
  - Impulses cannot be transmitted from atria to ventricle
- **AV dissociation**
  - Atria and ventricular depolarization uncoupled ("dissociated")
  - Can be caused by complete heart block
  - Also occurs if ventricular rate > sinus rate (no heart block)
  - Seen in ventricular tachycardia and other rhythms

Ventricular Tachycardia

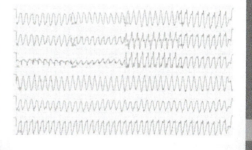

Ventricular Tachycardia

Escape Rhythm

- SA node: Dominant (fastest) pacemaker
- Heart block: SA cannot send impulses to ventricles
- Other pacemakers exist but are slower
  - SA node (60-100 bpm)
  - AV node (40-60 bpm)
  - HIS (25-40 bpm)
  - Bundle branches (25-40 bpm)
  - Purkinje fibers (25-40 bpm)

Escape Rhythm

- Heart block: lower pacemaker depolarizes ventricles
  - "Escape rhythm"
- Rate of lower pacemaker determines symptoms
  - Very slow: dizziness, syncope, hypotension
  - Less slow: fatigue, exercise intolerance

Sites of AV Block

Disorder	Common Site of Block
1st Degree	AV node
Mobitz I	AV Node
Mobitz II	His-Purkinje System
3rd degree (Complete)	His-Purkinje System

Causes of Heart Block

- Drugs
  - Beta blockers, calcium channel blockers
  - Digoxin
- High vagal tone
  - Athletes
- Fibrosis and sclerosis of conduction system

Pacemaker

- Treatment for "high grade" AV block
- Usually 3rd degree or Mobitz II
- Often in patients with symptoms (syncope, dizziness)

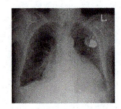 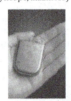

Bundle Branch Blocks

- Both bundle branches blocked
  - Results in AV block
  - Form of HIS-Purkinje system disease
- ONE bundle branch blocked
  - Does not cause AV block
  - Normal PR interval
  - QRS will be prolonged

Right Bundle Branch Block

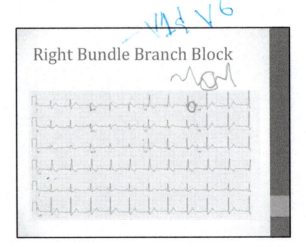

Left Bundle Branch Block

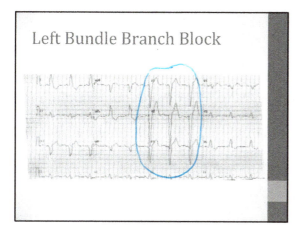

Bundle Branch Blocks

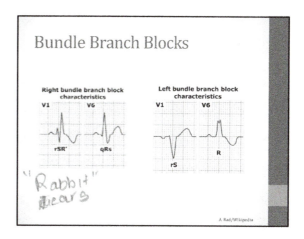

"Rabbit ears"

Bundle Branch Blocks

- Symptoms: None
  - Identified incidentally on ECG
- May progress to AV block (need for pacemaker)
- Interfere with detection of ischemia
  - ST elevations, T-wave inversions can be normal

Bundle Branch Blocks
Causes

- Often caused by slowly progressive fibrosis/sclerosis
- More common in older patients
- Can result from "structural heart disease"
- LBBB: Prior MI, cardiomyopathy
- RBBB: Right heart failure

"W" V6
"L" V6

Atrial Fibrillation and Flutter

Jason Ryan, MD, MPH

Atrial Fibrillation

- Cardiac arrhythmia
- Results in an irregularly, irregular pulse
- Diagnosis: EKG

Atrial Fibrillation

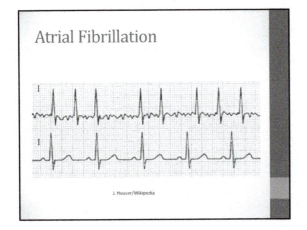

J. Heuser/Wikipedia

Atrial Fibrillation

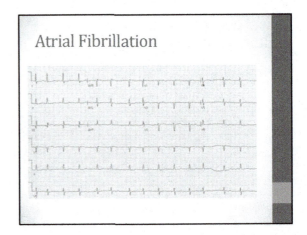

Atrial Fibrillation

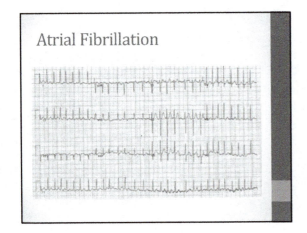

Atrial Fibrillation

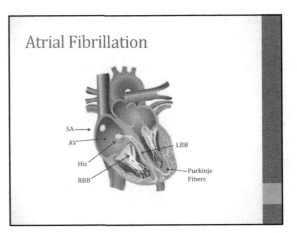

Atrial Fibrillation
Terminology

- Paroxysmal
  - Comes and goes; spontaneous conversion to sinus rhythm
- Persistent
  - Lasts days/weeks; often requires cardioversion
- Permanent

Atrial Fibrillation
Symptoms

- Wide spectrum of symptoms

⟷

Asymptomatic   Palpitations, Dyspnea, Fatigue
Heart Rate <100bpm   Heart Rate >100bpm

Cardiomyopathy

- Caused by untreated, **rapid** atrial fibrillation
- "Tachycardia-induced cardiomyopathy"
- ↓ LVEF
- Systolic heart failure

Heart Rate

- **AV node refractory period** determines heart rate
- Young, healthy patients → rapid heart rate
- Older patients → slower heart rate
- Atrial rate in fibrillation: 300-500bpm
- Ventricular rate: 70-180bpm

Preload

- Atrial fibrillation eliminates ventricular pre-filling
- "Loss of atrial kick"
- **Decreases preload**
- Can lead to low cardiac output and hypotension
- Especially in "preload dependent" patients
  - Aortic stenosis
  - LVH or diastolic heart failure (stiff ventricle)

Atrial Fibrillation
Thrombus in Left Atrial Appendage

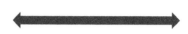

Atrial Fibrillation
Cardiac Embolism

- Brain (stroke)
- Gut (mesenteric ischemia)
- Spleen

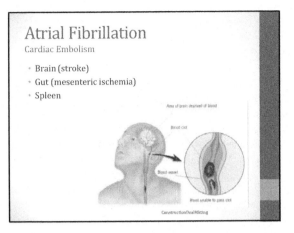

Valvular Atrial Fibrillation

- Associated with rheumatic heart disease
- Usually **mitral stenosis**
- Often refractory to treatment
- VERY high risk of thrombus
- Non-valvular: not associated with rheumatic disease

Atrial Fibrillation
Risk Factors

- **Age**
  - ~10% of patients >80
  - <1% of patients <55
- More common in women
- Most common associated disorders: HTN, CAD
- Anything that dilates the atria → atrial fibrillation
  - Heart failure
  - Valvular disease
- Key diagnostic test: Echocardiogram

Hyperthyroidism

- Commonly leads to atrial fibrillation
- Reversible with therapy for thyroid disease
- Atrial fibrillation therapies less effective
- Key diagnostic test: TSH

Atrial Fibrillation
Triggers

- Often no trigger identified
- Binge drinking ("holiday heart")
- Increased catecholamines
  - Infection
  - Surgery
  - Pain

Atrial Fibrillation
Treatment

- Heart Rate
  - "Rate control"
  - Ideally <110bpm
- Heart Rhythm
  - "Rhythm control"
  - Restoration of sinus rhythm
- Anticoagulation

Rate Control

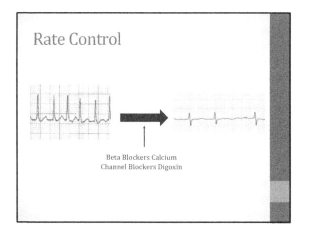

Beta Blockers Calcium
Channel Blockers Digoxin

Rate Control

- Use drugs that **slow AV node conduction**
- Beta blockers
  - Usually β1 selective agents
  - Metoprolol, Atenolol
- Calcium channel blockers
  - Verapamil, Diltiazem
- Digoxin
  - Increases parasympathetic tone to heart

Rhythm Control

- Goal: restore sinus rhythm

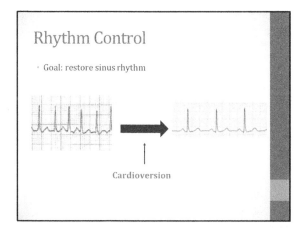

Cardioversion

Cardioversion

- **Electrical**
  - Deliver "synchronized" shock at time of QRS
  - Administer anesthesia
  - Deliver electrical shock to chest
  - All myocytes depolarize
  - Usually sinus node first to repolarize/depolarize

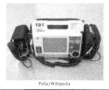

Pollo/Wikipedia

Cardioversion

- **Chemical**
  - Administration of antiarrhythmic medication
  - Often Ibutilide (class III antiarrhythmic)
  - Less commonly used due to drug toxicity

Cardioversion

- **Spontaneous**
  - Often occurs after hours/days

Cardioversion
Risk of Stroke

- Chemical/electrical cardioversion may cause stroke
- 48hours required for thrombus formation
- Symptoms <48hours: cardioversion safe
- Symptoms >48hours (or unsure)
  - Anti-coagulation 3 weeks → cardioversion
  - Transesophageal echocardiogram to exclude thrombus
- Exception: Hypotension/shock
  - Emergent cardioversion performed

Rhythm Control

- Antiarrhythmic medications
- Administered before/after cardioversion
- Class I drugs
  - Flecainide, propafenone
- Class III drugs
  - Amiodarone, sotalol, dofetilide

Anticoagulation

- Warfarin
  - Requires regular INR monitoring
  - Goal INR usually 2-3
- Rivaroxaban, Apixaban
  - Factor X inhibitors
- Dabigatran
  - Direct thrombin inhibitor
- Aspirin
  - Less effective
  - Only used if risk of stroke is very low
  - Less risk of bleeding

Anticoagulation

- Whether atrial fibrillation persists or sinus rhythm restored anticoagulation MUST be administered
- Studies show similar stroke risk for rate control versus rhythm control

Stroke Risk

- CHADS Score
  - CHF (1 point)
  - HTN (1 point)
  - Age >75yrs (1 point)
  - Diabetes (1 point)
  - Stroke (2 points)
- Score ≥2 = Warfarin or other anticoagulant
- Score 0 -1 = Aspirin

Stroke Risk

- CHADS VASC Score
  - CHF (1point)
  - HTN (1pont)
  - Diabetes (1point)
  - Stroke (2points)
  - Female (1point)
  - Age 65-75 (1point)
  - Age >75yrs (2points)
  - Vascular disease (1point)
- Score ≥2 = Warfarin or other anticoagulant
- Score 0 -1 = Aspirin

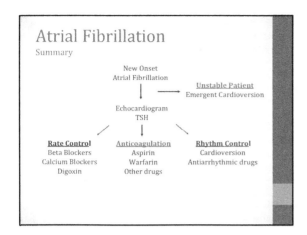
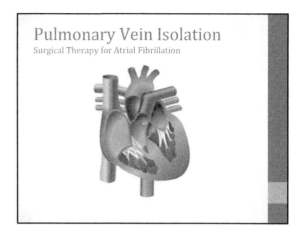
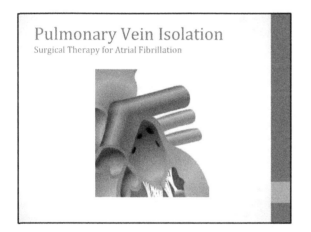
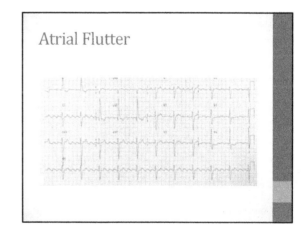
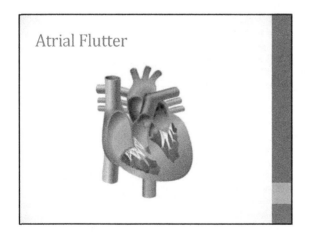

Atrial Flutter
Treatment

- Generally the same as atrial fibrillation
- Rate or rhythm control
- Rate-slowing drugs
- Cardioversion
- Anticoagulation based on stroke risk

Atrial Flutter Ablation

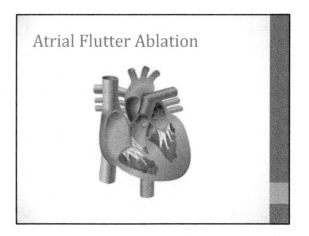

AVNRT

Jason Ryan, MD, MPH

PSVT
Paroxysmal Supraventricular Tachycardia

- Intermittent tachycardia (HR > 100bpm)
- **Sudden onset/offset**
  - Contrast with sinus tachycardia
- Electrical activity originates above ventricle
  - "Supraventricular"
  - Contrast with ventricular tachycardia
  - Produces narrow QRS complex (<120ms)

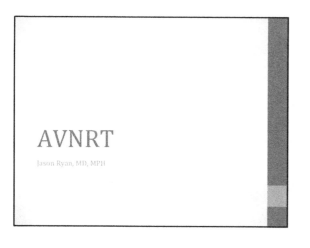

PSVT
Paroxysmal Supraventricular Tachycardia

- Often causes sudden-onset palpitations
- Chest discomfort
- Rarely syncope

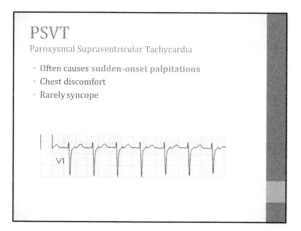

AVNRT
Atrioventricular nodal reentrant tachycardia

- Most common cause of PSVT
- More common in young women
- Mean age onset: 32 years old
- Requires **dual AV nodal pathways**

Normal Conduction

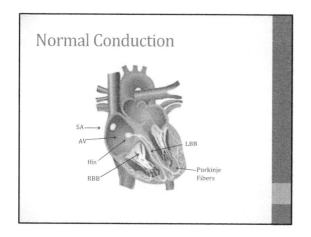

Dual Pathways
Sinus Rhythm

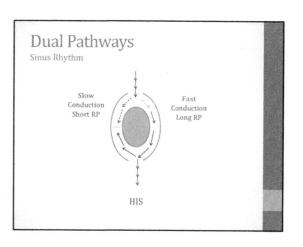

Dual Pathways
PAC

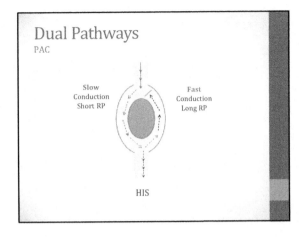

Retrograde P Waves

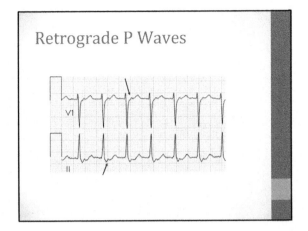

AVNRT

- Recurrent episodes of palpitations
- Many episodes spontaneously resolve
- ↓ conduction in AV node breaks arrhythmia
  - Will halt conduction is slow pathway
- Carotid massage
- Vagal maneuvers
- Adenosine

Carotid Massage

- Examiner presses on neck near carotid sinus
- Stretch of baroreceptors
- CNS response as if high blood pressure
- Increased vagal tone
- ↓ AV node conduction

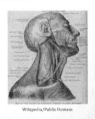

Wikipedia/Public Domain

Vagal Maneuvers

- Valsalva
  - Patient bears down as if moving bowels
  - Increased thoracic pressure
  - Aortic pressure rises → ↓ heart rate and AV conduction
- Breath holding
- Coughing
- Deep respirations
- Gagging
- Swallowing

AVNRT
Chronic Treatment

- Many patients need no therapy
- Beta blockers, Verapamil/Diltiazem
  - Slow conduction in slow pathway
- Surgical ablation of slow pathway

Wolff-Parkinson White

Jason Ryan, MD, MPH

WPW Syndrome
Wolff-Parkinson White Syndrome

- Cardiac electrical disorder
- "Accessory atrioventricular pathway"
  - Conducts impulses from atria to ventricles
  - Bypasses AV node
  - "Bundle of Kent"
  - Ventricular depolarization before AV nodal impulse
- May lead to **arrhythmias**

EKG in WPW

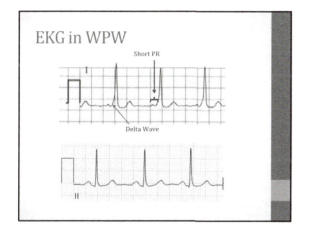

Short PR
Delta Wave

WPW EKG

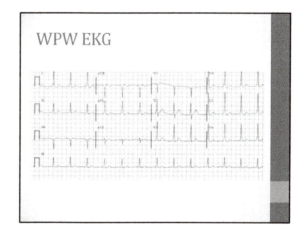

Cardiac Electrical System

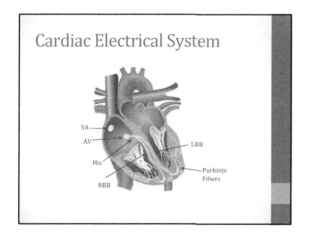

SA, AV, His, RBB, LBB, Purkinje Fibers

AVRT
AV Re-entrant Tachycardia

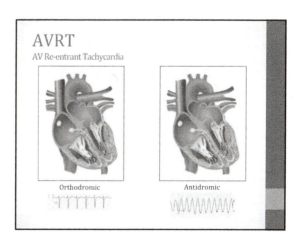

Orthodromic   Antidromic

Bypass Tract Consequences

- Most patients asymptomatic
  - EKG with delta wave only
  - Called WPW "pattern"
- Some have tachycardias
  - Presents as palpitations
  - Called **WPW syndrome**
  - AVRT (anti or orthodromic)
- Rarely causes syncope or sudden death
- Treatment: Ablation of accessory pathway

Atrial Fibrillation in WPW

- Atrial fibrillation can be life threatening
- Atrial depolarization rate 300-500/min
- AV node conducts <200/min
- Impulses may conduct rapidly over bypass tract

Wide complex, irregular, tachycardic

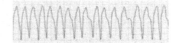

Atrial Fibrillation in WPW

- Slowing AV node conduction is dangerous
- Allows more impulses over bypass tract
- **Usual atrial fibrillation therapies contraindicated**
  - Beta blockers
  - Calcium channel blockers
  - Digoxin
  - Adenosine
- Acute treatment: Cardioversion or antiarrhythmics
  - Ibutilide, procainamide
  - Slow conduction in bypass tract

Antiarrhythmic Drugs

Jason Ryan, MD, MPH

Vaughan Williams

Class I		Class II
Quinidine / Procainamide	Ia	Beta Blockers
Lidocaine / Mexiletine	Ib	
Flecainide / Propafenone	Ic	

Class III	Class IV
Amiodarone, Sotalol, Dofetilide, Ibutilide	Ca-channel Blockers (Verapamil/Diltiazem)

Use of Antiarrhythmic Drugs

- Drugs used to "suppress" arrhythmias
- Prevent formation of aberrant impulses
- Most also *cause* arrhythmias
- Can lead to cardiac arrest and death
- Used in dangerous arrhythmias
- Also used in recurrent symptomatic arrhythmias

Use of Antiarrhythmic Drugs

- Persistent/recurrent ventricular tachycardia
- Recurrent atrial fibrillation

Ventricular Tachycardia

Rapid Atrial Fibrillation

Mechanisms

- All drugs slow cardiac electrical activity
- Class I drugs → Block Na channel
- Class III drugs → Block K channels
- Class II, IV: Slow sinus and AV node conduction

Class I, III   BB, CCB (Class II, IV)

Myocyte Action Potential
Atrial/ventricular myocytes

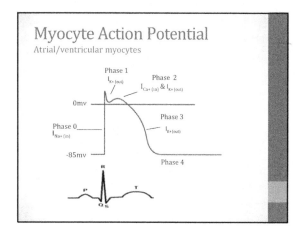

Na Channel Blockade

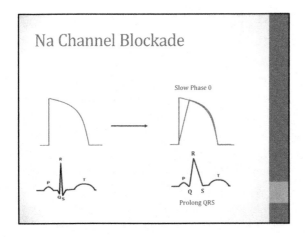

Slow Phase 0

Prolong QRS

K Channel Blockade

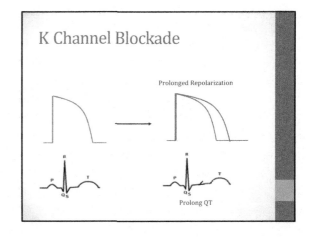

Prolonged Repolarization

Prolong QT

Myocyte Action Potential
Atrial/ventricular myocytes

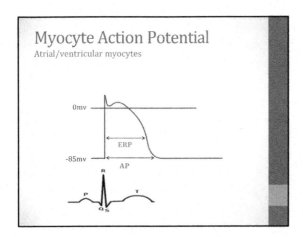

Class I drugs

- Block sodium channels → prolong QRS
- Some also affect K+ channels → prolong Qt
- Can prolong action potential duration
- Can prolong effective refractory period

Class I drugs
Effects on Resting Action Potential

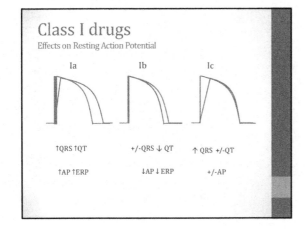

Ia	Ib	Ic
↑QRS ↑QT	+/-QRS ↓ QT	↑ QRS +/-QT
↑AP ↑ERP	↓AP ↓ERP	+/-AP

Class Ia Drugs
Quinidine, procainamide

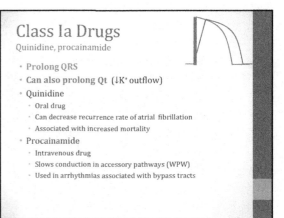

- **Prolong QRS**
- **Can also prolong Qt (↓K⁺ outflow)**
- Quinidine
  - Oral drug
  - Can decrease recurrence rate of atrial fibrillation
  - Associated with increased mortality
- Procainamide
  - Intravenous drug
  - Slows conduction in accessory pathways (WPW)
  - Used in arrhythmias associated with bypass tracts

Procainamide

- Associated with **drug-induced lupus**
  - Classic drugs: INH, hydralazine, procainamide
- Often rash, arthritis, anemia
- Antinuclear antibody (ANA) can be positive
- Key features: **anti-histone antibodies**
- Resolves on stopping the drug

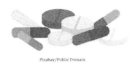
Pixabay/Public Domain

Class Ib Drugs
Lidocaine, Mexiletine

- Little/no effect on QRS at normal HR
- Slight decrease in Qt interval (minimal)
- **Least effect on action potential of class 1 drugs**

Class Ib Drugs
Lidocaine, Mexiletine

- Most Na channel binding in **depolarized state**
- Ischemia → more depolarized myocytes
- Effective drugs in ischemic arrhythmias

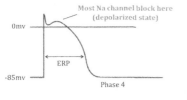

Class Ib Drugs
Lidocaine, Mexiletine

- **Drug rapidly unbinds**
- Slow heart rates: little drug effect by next heart beat
- More effective in fast heart rates
- Less time to unbind before Na channels open again
- Main use: ischemic ventricular tachycardia
  - Fast heart rates
  - Depolarized Na channels

Class Ib Drugs
Lidocaine, Mexiletine

- Lidocaine also a local anesthetic
  - Na channel nerve block
- May cause **CNS stimulation**
  - Tremor, agitation
  - Tremor in patient on Mexiletine = toxicity
- Cardiovascular side effects
  - From excessive block of Na channels
  - Bradycardia, heart block, hypotension

Class Ic Drugs
Flecainide, Propafenone

- Block open Na channels
- Very slow unbinding
- Result: QRS can markedly prolong
- Limited use due to concern of toxicity
- Especially proarrhythmic effects

CAST Trial
The Cardiac Arrhythmia Suppression Trial

- Landmark clinical trial of antiarrhythmic drugs
- Tested the suppression hypothesis
  - Suppression of arrhythmias with drugs is a good thing
- Patients with asymptomatic arrhythmias after MI
- Encainide and flecainide administered
- Patients taking drugs had less arrhythmias
- Also: **3.6-fold increased risk of arrhythmic death**
- Result: Major ↓ antiarrhythmic drugs
- Now used only with compelling indication

Class Ic Drugs
Flecainide, Propafenone

- Only used in patients with structurally normal hearts
- Effective in reducing recurrence of atrial fibrillation
- Must monitor for **QRS prolongation**
- Prolonged QRS → Risk of cardiac arrest

Use Dependence

- Na channels fluctuate between 3 different states
- Resting, Open and Inactivated
- Drugs bind more in certain states
- Class I drugs bind best in open/inactivate states
  - States when Na channel is in "use"
- These drug exhibit "use dependence"

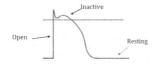

Use Dependence

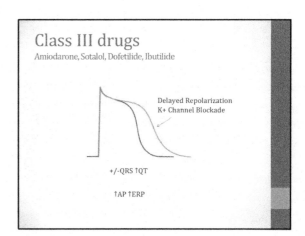

Use Dependence

- **Use dependent drugs: more binding fast heart rates**
- All class I drugs have some use dependence
- Seen most frequently IC drugs
- Practical implication:
  - Flecainide and propafenone (IC drugs)
  - Marked use dependence
  - Toxicity (QRS prolongation) at high heart rates
  - Stress testing often done to screen for toxicity

Class III drugs
Amiodarone, Sotalol, Dofetilide, Ibutilide

Delayed Repolarization
K+ Channel Blockade

+/- QRS ↑QT

↑AP ↑ERP

Torsade de Pointes

- Feared outcome of Qt prolongation
- Results in cardiac arrest
- Class IA, III drugs prolong Qt

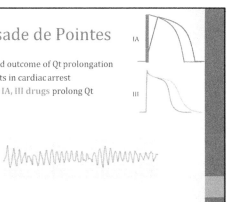

Amiodarone

- Class III drug
  - K channel blocker: Prolongs Qt interval
  - Lowest incidence TDP of all class IIIs
- Also has class I, II, and IV effects
  - Class I: Prolongs QRS
  - Class II, IV: Slow HR, delay AV conduction
- Very effective drug
- Suppresses atrial fibrillation
- Suppresses ventricular tachycardia

Amiodarone

- Highly lipid soluble
- Accumulates in liver, lungs, skin, other tissues
- Half-life about 58 days
- Once steady state reached, very long washout
- Safe in renal disease (biliary excretion)

Amiodarone

- Many potential side effects related to accumulation
- Less likely at lower dosages
- Risk accumulates over time
- Young patients on indefinite therapy at greatest risk
- Often used in older patients

Amiodarone
Side Effects

- **Hyper and hypothyroidism**
  - Contains iodine
- **Increased LFTs**
  - Usually asymptomatic and mild
  - Drug stopped if elevation is marked
- **Skin sensitivity to sun**
  - Patients easily sunburn

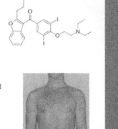

Wikipedia/Public Domain

Amiodarone
Side Effects

- **Blue-gray discoloration**
  - Less common skin reaction
  - "Blue man syndrome"
  - Most prominent on face
- Corneal deposits
  - Secretion of amiodarone by lacrimal glands
  - Accumulation on corneal surface
  - Appearance of "cat whiskers" on cornea
  - Does not usually cause vision problems
  - See in many patients on chronic therapy

Amiodarone
Side Effects

- Pulmonary fibrosis
- Most common cause of death from amiodarone
- Foamy macrophages seen in air spaces
- Filled with amiodarone and phospholipids
- "Honeycombing" pattern on chest x-ray

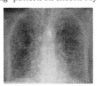

Amiodarone
Side Effects

- When starting amiodarone
  - Chest X-ray
  - Pulmonary function tests (PFTs)
  - Thyroid function tests (TFTs)
  - Liver function tests (LFTs)

Sotalol and Dofetilide

- Both drugs block K channels (class III)
- Can prolong Qt interval → torsade de pointes
- Practical consideration:
  - Patients often admitted to hospital to start therapy
  - Rhythm monitored on telemetry
  - Qt segment checked by EKG each day
- Sotalol: Also has beta blocking properties
- Can be used in patients with cardiomyopathy
- "Reverse use dependence"

Reverse Use Dependence

- K channels also fluctuate between 3 different states
- Class III drugs bind best in resting state
- These drug exhibit "reverse use dependence"

Reverse Use Dependence

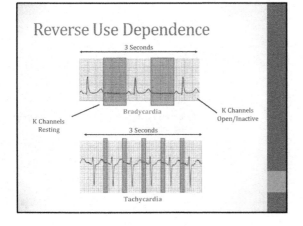

Sotalol and Dofetilide

- Reverse use dependence: more binding slow rates
- Practical implication:
  - Bradycardia in patient on sotalol/dofetilide
  - Qt interval may prolong
  - Increased risk of torsade de pointes

Sotalol and Dofetilide

- Commonly used in patients with **atrial fibrillation**
- Typical case
  - Recurrent episodes symptomatic atrial fibrillation
  - Sotalol/Dofetilide started
  - Cardioversion to restore sinus rhythm
  - Sinus rhythm persists on therapy
- Other antiarrhythmic also used in this manner
  - Amiodarone
  - Propafenone
  - Flecainide

Ibutilide

- Intravenous drug
- Half life of 2 to 12 hours
- Used for "chemical cardioversion"

Cardioversion

- Termination of arrhythmias
- Often atrial fibrillation or flutter

Electrical Cardioversion
Requires sedation

Chemical Cardioversion
No sedation   May cause Torsade

Ibutilide

Beta Blockers
Class II Antiarrhythmics

- Main effect: **Pacemaker cells (SA and AV node)**
- Decrease slope of phase 4
- Prolong repolarization (phase 3)

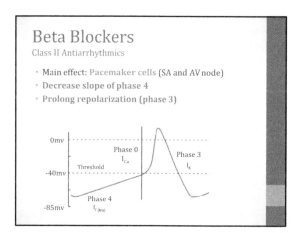

Beta Blockers
Class II Antiarrhythmics

↓HR
↓Cond Velocity
↑PR Interval

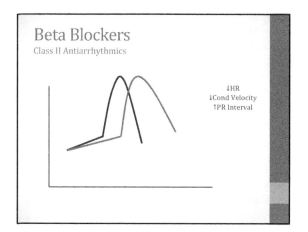

Calcium Channel Blockers
Verapamil and Diltiazem

- Block calcium channels
- Slow heart rate
- Slow AV node conduction

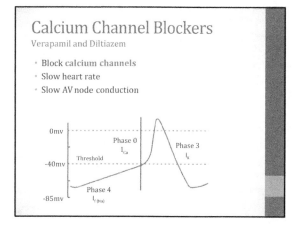

Calcium Channel Blockers
Verapamil and Diltiazem

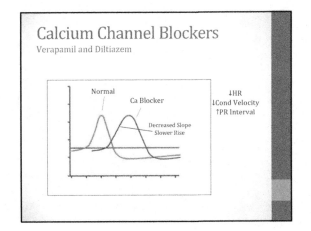

↓HR
↓Cond Velocity
↑PR Interval

AV Block

- Beta blockers/Ca channel blockers → ↓ AV conduction

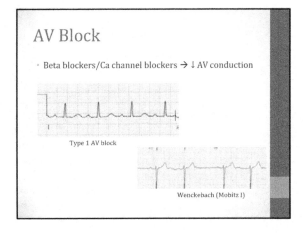

Type 1 AV block

Wenckebach (Mobitz I)

Atrial Fibrillation

- Beta blockers and CCBs commonly used
- Control ventricular rate

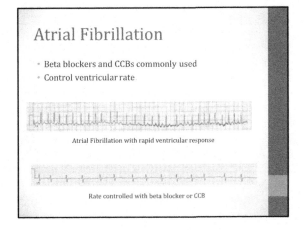

Atrial Fibrillation with rapid ventricular response

Rate controlled with beta blocker or CCB

Sudden Cardiac Death

- Increased risk among systolic heart failure patients
- Lower rates among patients on beta blockers
- Improved mortality

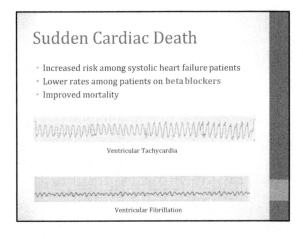

Ventricular Tachycardia

Ventricular Fibrillation

Adenosine

- Nucleoside base
- Used to make ATP
- Receptors in many locations (purinergic receptors)
  - AV nodal tissue
  - Vascular smooth muscle

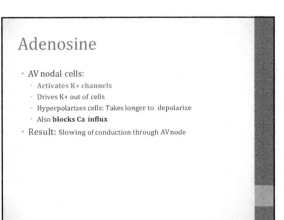

Adenosine Triphosphate

Adenosine

- AV nodal cells:
  - Activates K+ channels
  - Drives K+ out of cells
  - Hyperpolarizes cells: Takes longer to depolarize
  - Also **blocks Ca influx**
- Result: Slowing of conduction through AV node

Adenosine

- Short half life
- Given IV for acute therapy of SVT
- Slows AV node conduction

Narrow Complex
Originates above HIS bundle

Adenosine

- Most common SVT: **AVNRT**
  - AV node reentrant tachycardia
- Slow and fast circuits in AV node → arrhythmia
- Adenosine slows AV node conduction
- Arrhythmia with terminate

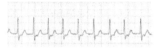

Adenosine

- Effects blocked by **theophylline** and **caffeine**
- Block adenosine receptors

Adenosine   Caffeine   Theophylline

Adenosine

- Also a vasodilator
- Causes skin flushing, hypotension
- Some patients also develop dyspnea, chest pain
- Effects quickly resolve
- Must warn patients before administration for SVT

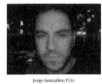

Jorge González/Flikr

Magnesium

- Acute management of **torsade de pointes**
- Mg blocks influx of Ca into cells
- Ca influx leads to early afterdepolarizations

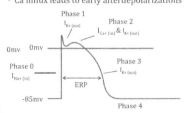

Atropine

- Muscarinic receptor antagonist
  - Parasympathetic block → ↑ HR and AV conduction
- Used in bradycardia → ↑ heart rate
- Also speeds conduction through AV node
- Useful for bradycardia especially from AV block

Atropine

Before Atropine

After Atropine

Atropine

- May side effects related to muscarinic block
- Toxicity:
  - Dry mouth
  - Constipation
  - Urinary retention
  - Confusion (elderly)

Digoxin

- Two cardiac effects
- #1: Increases contractility
  - Used in systolic heart failure with ↓ LVEF
- #2: Slows AV node conduction
  - Used in atrial fibrillation to slow ventricular rate

Digoxin
Increased Contractility

- Inhibits Na-K-ATPase

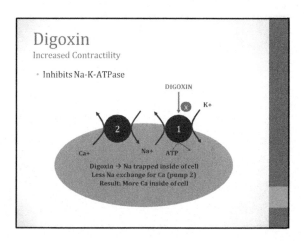

Digoxin
AV Nodal Slowing

- **Suppresses AV node conduction**
  - Increased **vagal (parasympathetic) tone**
  - Separate effect from blockade of Na-K-ATPase
- Can be used to ↓ **heart rate** in rapid atrial fibrillation
  - Continued atrial fibrillation
  - Fewer impulses to ventricle → slower heart rate
- Effects similar to BB and CCB in AV node

Digoxin Toxicity

- **Renal** clearance
  - Risk of toxicity in patients with chronic kidney disease
- **Hypokalemia** promotes toxicity
  - Caused by many diuretics, especially loop diuretics
  - Digoxin patient on furosemide → toxicity
- Levels often need to be monitored

Digoxin Toxicity

- Gastrointestinal
  - Anorexia, nausea, vomiting, abdominal pain
- Neurologic
  - Lethargy, fatigue
  - Delirium, confusion, disorientation
  - Weakness
- Visual changes
  - Alterations in color vision, scotomas, blindness
- Cardiac arrhythmias

Digoxin Toxicity
Cardiac Toxicity

- More Na inside of cell
- ↑ resting potential atrial/ventricular cells
- Increased automaticity
- Dig toxic rhythms:
  - Extra beats: atrial, junctional, ventricular
  - Evidence of AV node block

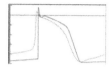

Digoxin Toxicity
Treatment

- Digibind
  - Digoxin antigen binding fragments (Fab)
  - Produced in animals (sheep)
  - Dig bound to albumin (hapten) → antibodies
  - Antibody converted to fragments
- Corrects hyperkalemia, symptoms

Heart Murmurs

Jason Ryan, MD, MPH

Heart Murmurs

- Cardiac sound heard with stethoscope
- Caused by turbulent blood flow
- May be normal or pathologic

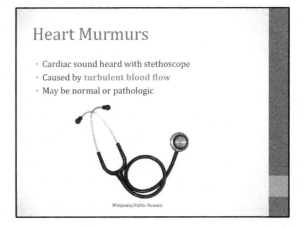

Wikipedia/Public Domain

Laminar vs. Turbulent Flow

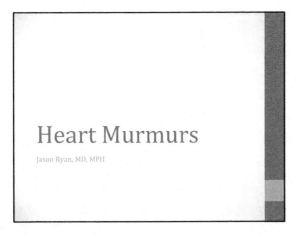

Laminar Flow = Quiet(er)

Turbulent Flow = Loud
High Flow Rates
Narrow Flow Areas

Murmurs
Grading

- I - barely audible on listening carefully
- II - faint but easily audible
- III - loud and easily audible, no thrill
- IV - loud murmur with a thrill
- V - heard with scope barely touching chest
- VI - audible with scope not touching the chest

Murmurs
Other Descriptors

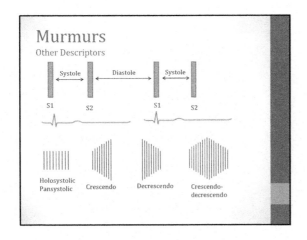

Holosystolic/Pansystolic, Crescendo, Decrescendo, Crescendo-decrescendo

Murmurs
Location

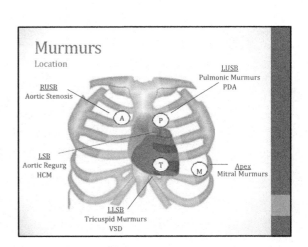

- RUSB: Aortic Stenosis
- LUSB: Pulmonic Murmurs, PDA
- LSB: Aortic Regurg, HCM
- LLSB: Tricuspid Murmurs, VSD
- Apex: Mitral Murmurs

Murmurs
Location

- Point of maximal impulse (apical impulse)
  - Left 5th intercostal space
  - Mid-clavicular line
- Lateral shift = Enlarged heart
- Hyperdynamic

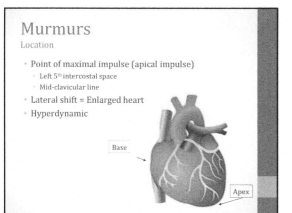

Innocent/Functional Murmurs

- Caused by normal flow of blood
- Common in children
- Also young, thin patients
- Generally soft murmurs
- No signs/symptoms of heart disease
- Stills murmur
- Pulmonic flow murmur
- Venous hum

Systolic Murmurs

- Occur when heart contracts/squeezes
- Between S1-S2
- Aortic stenosis
- Mitral regurgitation
- Pulmonic stenosis
- Tricuspid regurgitation
- Hypertrophic cardiomyopathy
- Ventricular septal defect (VSD)

Diastolic Murmurs

- Occur when heart relaxes/fills
- Between S2-S1
- Aortic regurgitation
- Mitral stenosis
- Pulmonic regurgitation
- Tricuspid stenosis

Aortic Stenosis
Murmur

- Systolic crescendo-decrescendo murmur
- Also called an "ejection murmur"

S1   S2

Aortic Stenosis
Severe Disease Findings

- Late-peaking murmur
  - Slow flow across stenotic valve
- Soft/quiet S2
  - Stiff valve can't slam shut
- **Pulsus parvus et tardus**
  - Weak and small carotid pulses
  - Delayed carotid upstroke

HCM
Hypertrophic Cardiomyopathy

- Same murmur as aortic stenosis
- Differentiated by maneuvers
- Valsalva
  - Decreases venous return/preload
  - Increase HCM murmur
  - Decrease AS murmur

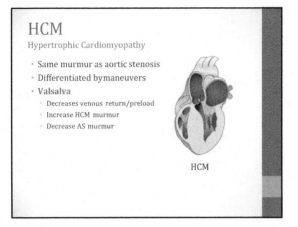

HCM

Aortic Regurgitation
Murmur

- Decrescendo, **blowing** diastolic murmur

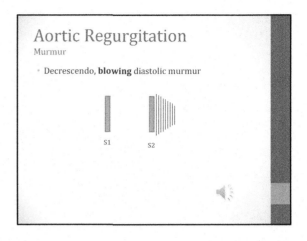

Mitral Regurgitation

- **Holosystolic murmur heard best at the apex**
  - 5th intercostal space, mid-clavicular line

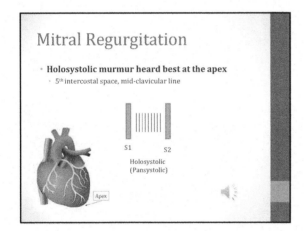

Mitral Stenosis

- **Diastolic rumbling murmur**
- Preceded by **opening snap**

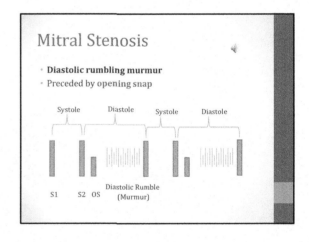

Mitral Stenosis

- No left sided S3, S4 in mitral stenosis
- **Time to opening snap** associated with severity
  - High left atrial pressure in severe disease
  - Higher left atrial pressure → ↓ time to opening snap
  - Short time to opening snap seen in severe disease

Tricuspid/Pulmonic Disease

- Valve lesions sound like left sided-counterparts
- Heard in different locations
- Left upper sternal border
  - Pulmonic stenosis/regurgitation
- Left lower sternal border
  - Tricuspid stenosis/regurgitation

Carvallo's Sign

- Most right sided murmurs louder with inspiration
- Inspiration draws blood volume to lungs
- Louder right sided murmurs
- Softer left sided murmurs
- rIght sided murmurs increase with Inspiration
- lEft sided murmurs increase with Exhalation

VSD
Ventricular Septal Defect

- Holosystolic murmur similar to MR
- Small VSD → more turbulence → loud murmur

3 Causes Holosytolic Murmurs
- Mitral Regurgitation
- Tricuspid Regurgitation
- VSD

Holosystolic (Pansystolic)

PDA
Patent Ductus Arteriosus

- Continuous, "machine-like" murmur

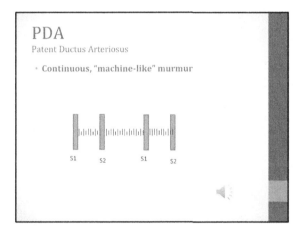

Maneuvers

- Performed at bedside with patient
- May increase or decrease murmur
- Used to make diagnosis

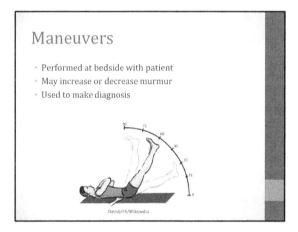

Maneuvers
Preload/Venous Return

- Increase preload/venous return
  - Leg raise – blood falls back toward heart
  - Squatting – blood in legs forced back toward heart
- Decrease preload/venous return
  - Valsalva- ↑ intra-thoracic pressure→ vein compression →↓ VR
  - Standing – Blood falls toward feet, away from heart
- Most murmurs INCREASE with more preload except:
  - HCM
  - MVP

Valsalva Maneuver

- Bear down as if moving bowels
- Phase I (few seconds)
  - ↑ thoracic pressure
  - ↓ venous return (compression of veins → ↑RA pressure)
  - Transient rise in aortic pressure (compression)
  - ↓ heart rate and AV node conduction (baroreceptors)
- Phase II
  - ↓ preload → ↓ cardiac output
  - ↑ heart rate and AV node conduction (baroreceptors)

Maneuvers
Afterload

- Increase Afterload
  - Hand grip - clench fist
- Decrease Afterload
  - Amyl Nitrate - vasodilator

Amyl Nitrate

Maneuvers
Afterload

- Backward Valve Disorders
  - AR, MR, VSD
  - Louder with more afterload
  - More force pushing blood backward
- Forward Valve Disorders
  - MS, AS
  - Softer with more afterload
  - Less pressure difference moving blood forward
- MVP, HCM
  - Softer
  - Increased LV cavity size

Clues to Diagnosis

- Young female, otherwise healthy → MVP
- Healthy, young athlete, syncope → HCM
- Immigrant or pregnant → Mitral stenosis
- IV drug abuser → Tricuspid regurgitation
- Turner Syndrome or Aortic Coarctation
  - Bicuspid AV
  - Early stenosis
  - Aortic regurgitation
- Marfan → MVP

Summary
Commonly Tested Murmurs

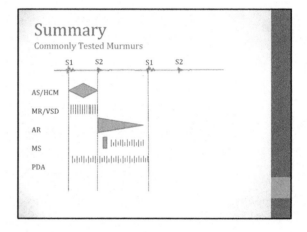

Heart Sounds

Jason Ryan, MD, MPH

The Cardiac Cycle

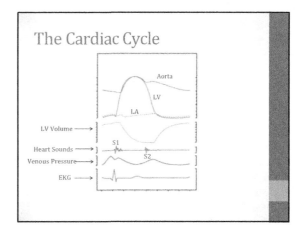

S1 and S2

- Normal heart sounds
- Each has two components
  - One from left sided valves (aortic, mitral)
  - One from right sided valves (tricuspid, pulmonic)
- S1 usually "single"
  - Two components close together
  - Cannot distinguish separate sounds
- S2 can be "split"
  - Two components far enough apart to be audible

S1 and S2

- S1
  - Mitral and tricuspid valves close
- S2
  - Aortic and pulmonary valves close

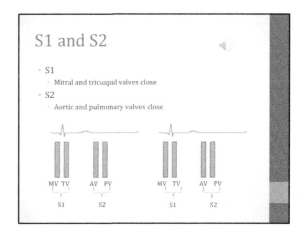

Physiologic S2 splitting

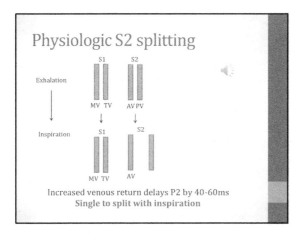

Increased venous return delays P2 by 40-60ms
Single to split with inspiration

Persistent S2 splitting
RBBB or Pulmonary Hypertension

PeRsistent = Right sided delay

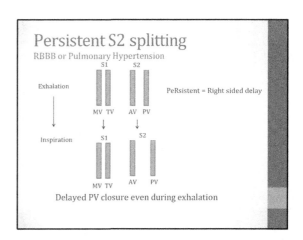

Delayed PV closure even during exhalation

Fixed S2 splitting
Atrial septal defect

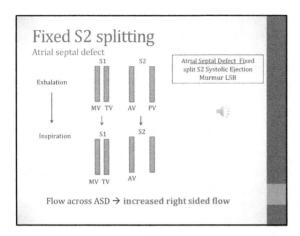

Flow across ASD → increased right sided flow

Paradoxical S2 splitting
Delayed closure of aortic valve

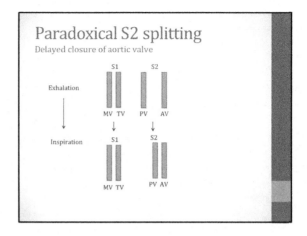

Paradoxical Splitting

- Electrical causes → delayed LV activation
  - LBBB
  - RV pacing
- Mechanical causes → delayed LV outflow
  - LV systolic failure
  - Aortic stenosis
  - Hypertrophic cardiomyopathy

ParodoxicaL = Left sided delay

Summary of S2 Splitting

- Physiologic = normal respiratory variation
- PeRsistent = RBBB, pulmonary HTN
- Fixed = Atrial septal defect
- ParadoxicaL = LBBB, cardiomyopathy

Cardiac Phonography

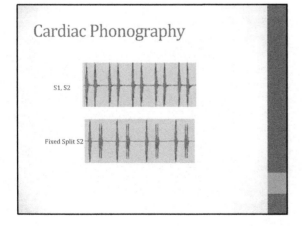

Loud P2

- Loud pulmonic component of S2
- **Pulmonary hypertension**
- Forceful closure of pulmonary valve
- Normally P2 not heard at apex
  - If you hear it here, it's "loud"

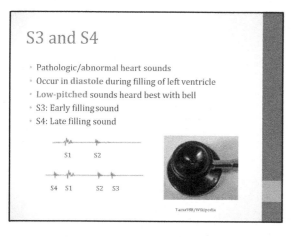
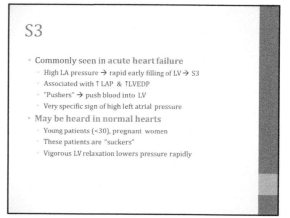
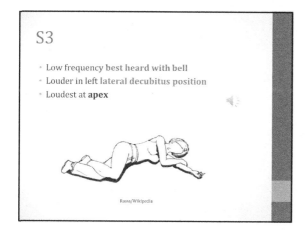
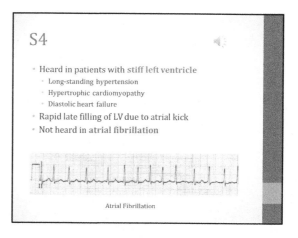
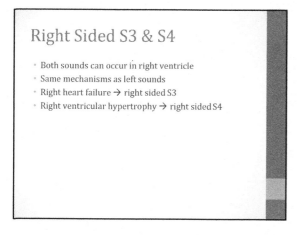
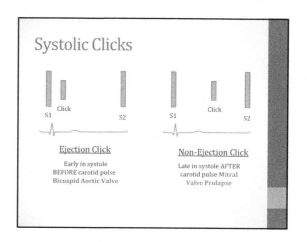

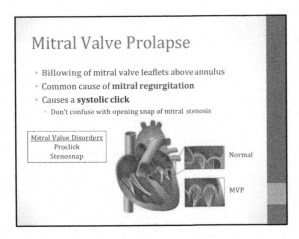
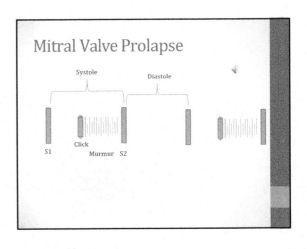

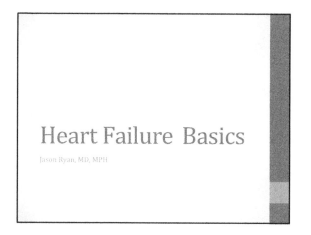
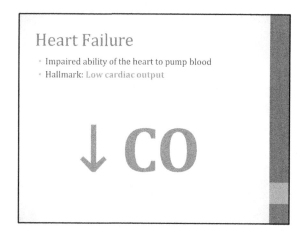
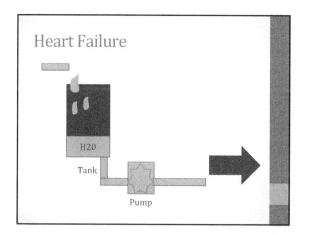
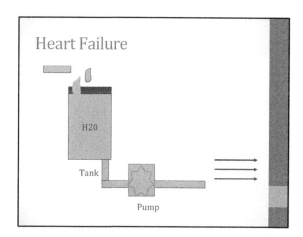
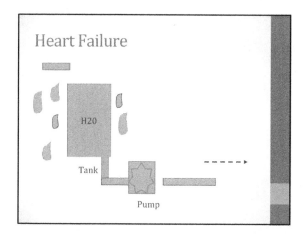
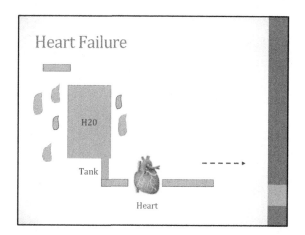

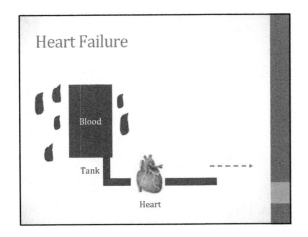
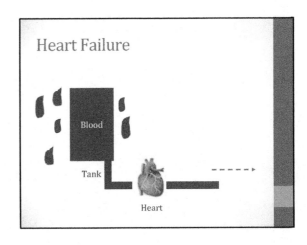
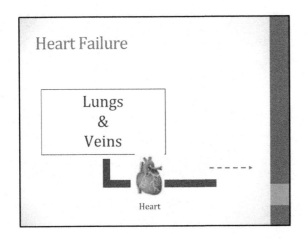

Heart Failure
Pathophysiology

- "Failing" chambers → Increased pressures
- Pressures rise in cardiac chambers

Heart Failure
Pathophysiology

- Left ventricular failure → ↑LV pressure
  - LV systolic pressure: depends on contractility (can be low)
  - LVEDP = always **high** in left heart failure
  - Hallmark of left heart failure
  - Less blood pumped out → more left behind → more pressure
  - Stiff ventricle (diastolic HF) → high pressure

Heart Failure
Pathophysiology

- ↑ LVEDP → ↑ LA pressure
- ↑ pulmonary capillary pressure
  - Dyspnea
  - **Pulmonary edema**

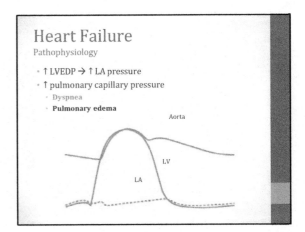

Heart Failure
Pathophysiology

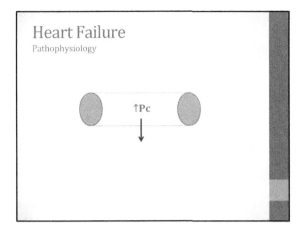

Heart Failure
Pathophysiology

- ↑ pulmonary capillary pressure → ↑ PA pressure
- ↑ PA pressure → ↑ RV pressure
- ↑ RV pressure → ↑ RA pressure
  - Right atrial pressure = central venous pressure
  - High pressure in venous system
  - ↑ jugular venous pressure (neck veins)
  - **Capillary leak → pitting edema**

Heart Failure
Signs/Symptoms

- Physiologic effects of lying flat (supine)
  - Increased venous return
  - Redistribution of blood volume
  - From lower extremities and splanchnic beds to lungs
- Little effect in normal individuals
- Impaired ventricle cannot tolerate changes
- Worsens pulmonary congestion and breathing

Heart Failure
Signs/Symptoms

- Left heart failure
  - Dyspnea especially on exertion
  - Paroxysmal nocturnal dyspnea (wake up SOB)
  - Orthopnea (can't breathe lying flat)
- Right heart failure
  - Increased jugular venous pressure
  - Lower extremity edema
  - Liver congestion (rarely can cause cirrhosis)
- "Backward failure"

Heart Failure
Right Heart Failure

- Most common cause R heart failure: Left heart failure
- Occasionally right heart failure occurs in isolation
  - Normal left atrial pressure
  - High pulmonary artery, right ventricular, right atrial pressure
  - Usually secondary to a lung process
  - Pulmonary hypertension
  - COPD
  - This is often called "cor pulmonale"

Heart Failure
Signs/Symptoms

- Low flow signs/symptoms ("forward failure")
  - Loss of appetite
  - Weight loss (cachexia)
  - Confusion
  - Cool extremities
  - "Narrow pulse pressure"
- Seen only with very low cardiac output (systolic HF)
- Not seen in diastolic heart failure

Heart Failure
Lung Findings

- Classic finding is **rales**
  - Fluid filled alveoli "pop" open with inspiration
- Chest X-ray shows congestion
- Lungs/CXR can be clear in chronic heart failure
  - ↑lymphatic drainage

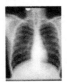 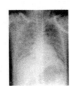

Heart Failure
Lung Findings

- Heart failure cells
- Hemosiderin (iron) laden macrophages
- Brown pigment in macrophages

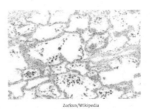

Zorkun/Wikipedia

Heart Failure
Signs/Symptoms

- Elevated **jugular venous pressure** (normal 6-8cmH2O)
- Look for height of double bounce (cause by a and v waves)

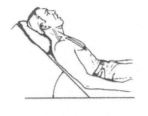

Heart Failure
Hepatojugular Reflux

- Pressure on abdomen raises JVP 1-3cm normally
- With failing RV, increase is greater

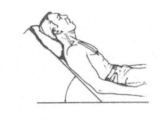

Heart Failure
Signs/Symptoms

- **Lower extremity pitting edema**
- Increased capillary hydrostatic pressure
- Fluid leak from capillaries → tissues
- Gravity pulls fluid to lower extremities

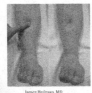 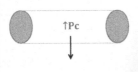

↑Pc

James Heilman, MD

Heart Failure
Abnormal Heart Sounds

- S3 (associated with high left atrial pressure)
- S4 (associated with stiff left ventricle)
- Displaced apical impulse – enlarged heart

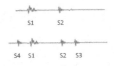

Heart Failure
Pathophysiology

- All forms of heart failure lead to ↓ cardiac output
- Activates two physiologic systems
  - Activation of **sympathetic nervous system**
  - Activation of **renin-angiotensin-aldosterone system**
  - All RAAS hormone levels will rise
- Both systems lead to two key effects:
  - Increased peripheral vascular resistance (vasoconstriction)
  - Retention of sodium/water (kidneys)

Heart Failure
Total Peripheral Resistance

- Cardiac output falls → vasoconstriction
- Angiotensin II, sympathetic nervous system
- **TPR always high**
- Blood pressure often high but may be low
- Depends on combined changes CO and TPR

$$BP = CO \times TPR$$

Heart Failure
Sodium/Water Retention

↓ cardiac output
↓
↓ Effective Circulating Volume
↓
↑RAAS ↑SNS ↑ADH
↓
↑ Na/H2O
↓
↑ Total Body Water

Heart Failure
Other Hormones

- **ANP (Atrial natriuretic peptide)**
- Atrial stretch (pressure/volume) → ANP release
- Vasodilator (↓TPR)
- Constricts renal efferents/dilates afferents
- ↑ diuresis
- Opposite effects of RAAS system

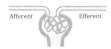

Heart Failure
Other Hormones

- ANP released by atrial myocytes
- **BNP (brain natriuretic peptide):** Ventricles
- Both rise with volume/pressure overload
- Both counter effects of RAAS system
- BNP sometimes used for diagnosis in dyspnea
  - High levels suggest heart failure
  - Low levels suggest other causes of dyspnea

RAAS — ANP/BNP

Nesiritide

- Recombinant BNP
- Vasodilation
- ↓ afterload, ↑CO
- Failed to show benefit in clinical trials

Heart Failure
Diagnosis

- Most common: typical signs/symptoms
- Elevated BNP level
- **Heart catheterization**
  - Increased LVEDP = left heart congestion/failure
  - Increased RA, RVEDP = right heart congestion/failure

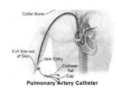

Systolic and Diastolic Heart Failure

Jason Ryan, MD, MPH

Heart Failure
Systolic and Diastolic

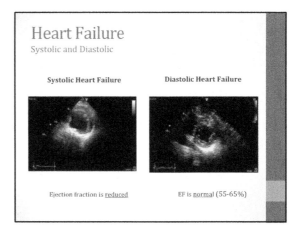

Systolic Heart Failure — Ejection fraction is reduced

Diastolic Heart Failure — EF is normal (55-65%)

Heart Failure
Systolic and Diastolic

- Same congestive signs/symptoms
  - Dyspnea, orthopnea, paroxysmal nocturnal dyspnea
  - Rales, ↑ JVP, pitting edema
- Exception: **Low flow symptoms** in systolic only
  - Cool extremities
  - Cachexia
  - Confusion

Dilated Cardiomyopathy

- Systolic heart failure with LV cavity dilation
- **"Eccentric" hypertrophy**
  - Volume overload (chronic retention of fluid in cavity)
  - Longer myocytes
  - Sarcomeres added in series

Normal LV Size → Dilated LV

Increased myocyte size
Sarcomeres in series
Normal wall thickness

Concentric Hypertrophy

- Pressure overload
- Chronic ↑↑ pressure in ventricle: HTN, Aortic stenosis
- Decreased compliance (stiff ventricle)
- Often seen in diastolic heart failure

Normal LV Size → ↓ LV Size

Increased myocyte size
Sarcomeres in parallel
Increased wall thickness

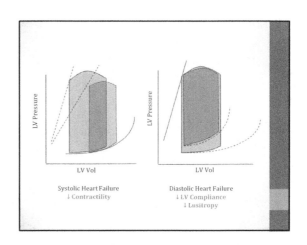

Systolic Heart Failure
↓ Contractility

Diastolic Heart Failure
↓ LV Compliance
↓ Lusitropy

Systolic Heart Failure

- ↓ Cardiac output
- Problem in SYSTOLE
- Can't get blood out
- ↓ Stroke volume
  - SV = EDV − ESV
  - ↑↑ ESV (↓ contractility)
  - ↑ EDV (↑ESV + VR)
  - ↑ LVEDP

Systolic Heart Failure
↓ Contractility

Frank-Starling Curve

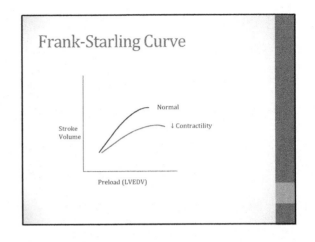

Diastolic Heart Failure

- ↓ Cardiac output
- Problem in DIASTOLE
- Can't get blood in
- Small ↓ stroke volume
  - ↓ EDV (↓ filling)
- ↑↑ LVEDP (stiff ventricle)

Diastolic Heart Failure
↓ LV Compliance
↓ Lusitropy

Systolic vs. Diastolic

	Normal	Systolic/Dilated	Diastolic
EDV	100	200	90
ESV	40	160	40
SV/CO	60	40	50
EF %	60	20	56

Systolic Heart Failure

- Most common cause: **Myocardial infarction**
  - Myocytes replaced by scar tissue
  - "Ischemic" cardiomyopathy
- Many causes of "non-ischemic" cardiomyopathy
  - About 50% idiopathic
  - Many other causes: viral, familial, peri-partum, chemotherapy toxicity, HIV, alcoholic, sarcoidosis, tachycardia-mediated

Diastolic Heart Failure

- Exact cause unknown
- Many cases have **concentric hypertrophy**
- Many associated conditions
  - Age, diabetes, hypertension
- Terms:
  - Heart failure preserved EF
  - HFpEF
  - Diastolic dysfunction

Nonischemic Cardiomyopathy
Viral

- May follow upper respiratory infection
- Many associated viruses
  - Coxsackie
  - Influenza, adenovirus, others
- Virus enters myocytes
- Causes myocarditis → cardiomyopathy
- Myocarditis phase may go undiagnosed
- No specific therapy for virus

Nonischemic Cardiomyopathy
Peri-partum

- Late in pregnancy or early post-pregnancy
- Exact cause unknown (likely multifactorial)
- Women often advised to avoid future pregnancy

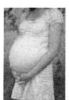

Nonischemic Cardiomyopathy
Chemotherapy

- Usually after treatment with anthracyclines
  - Antitumor antibiotics
  - Doxorubicin and daunorubicin

Daunorubicin

Doxorubicin (Adriamycin)

Nonischemic Cardiomyopathy
Familial

- Mutations
  - Often sarcomere proteins
  - Beta myosin heavy chain
  - Alpha myosin heavy chain
  - Troponin
- Many autosomal dominant
- X-linked, autosomal recessive also described

Nonischemic Cardiomyopathy
Tachycardia-mediated

- Constant, rapid heart rate for weeks/months
- Leads to depression of LV systolic function
- **Reversible** with slower heart rate

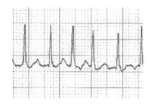

Nonischemic Cardiomyopathy
Takotsubo/Apical ballooning

- Stress-induced cardiomyopathy
- Occurs after severe emotional distress
- Markedly reduced LVEF
- Increase CK, MB, Troponin; EKG changes
- Looks like anterior MI (but no coronary disease)
- Usually recovers 4-6 weeks

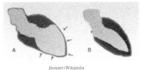

Alcohol

- Chronic consumption can cause cardiomyopathy
- Believed to be due to toxic metabolites
- Can recover with cessation of alcohol

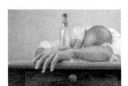

High Output Heart Failure

- Heart in overdrive
  - Severe anemia
  - Thyroid disease
  - Thiamine (B1) vitamin deficiency (beriberi)
  - A-V fistulas (post-surgical)
- Exact mechanism unclear
  - Decreased LV filling time
- Defining characteristic: HIGH cardiac output
  - Heart failure symptoms in absence of low output
  - ↑JVP, pulmonary edema

Restrictive Cardiomyopathy

Jason Ryan, MD, MPH

Restrictive Heart Disease

- Something "infiltrates" the myocardium
  - Granulomas (Sarcoid)
  - Amyloid protein (Amyloidosis)
- Heart cannot relax and fill
- SEVERE diastolic dysfunction

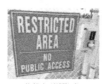

MarkBuckawicki/Wikipedia

Restrictive Heart Disease

- LVEF = normal
- Left ventricular volume = normal (not dilated)
- Restricted filling = ↑ atrial pressure
- Dilated left and right atria
- Classic imaging findings:
  - Normal left ventricular function/size
  - Bi-atrial enlargement

Restrictive Heart Disease
Clinical Features

- Dyspnea
- Prominent **right heart failure**
  - Markedly elevated jugular venous pressure
  - Lower extremity edema
  - Liver congestion
  - May lead to cirrhosis ("nutmeg liver")

David Monniaux/Wikipedia

Restrictive Heart Disease
Classic signs

- Kussmaul's sign
  - Inspiration causes rise in JVP

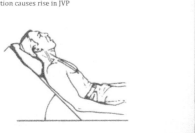

Restrictive Heart Disease
Rhythm Disturbances

- Myocardial infiltration may disrupt electrical activity
- Arrhythmias (sudden death)
- AV block

Ventricular Tachycardia   3rd Degree Heart Block

Restrictive Heart Disease
Major Causes

- Amyloidosis
  - Amyloid protein deposits in heart
  - Various forms (primary, secondary, etc.)

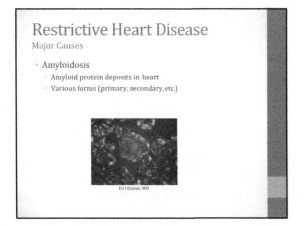

Restrictive Heart Disease
Classic signs

- Can see thickened myocardium
- Low voltage on EKG
- Classic finding in amyloidosis and Fabry's disease

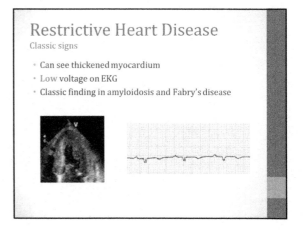

Restrictive Heart Disease
Major Causes

- Sarcoidosis
  - Granuloma formation
  - Usually involves lungs
  - Extra-pulmonary organs include heart

Restrictive Heart Disease
Major Causes

- **Fabry disease**
  - Lysosomal storage disease
  - Deficiency of α-galactosidase A
  - Accumulation of ceramide trihexoside

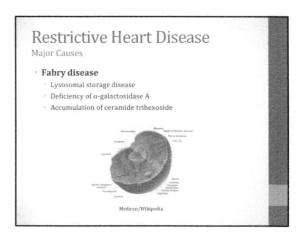

Restrictive Heart Disease
Major Causes

- **Hemochromatosis**
  - **Iron** excess
  - Commonly causes dilated cardiomyopathy
  - Rarely may cause restrictive

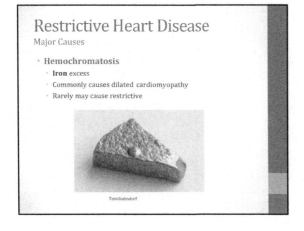

Restrictive Heart Disease
Major Causes

- Post-radiation
- Acutely: May cause inflammation
- Fibroblast recruitment
- **Extra-cellar matrix deposition**
- Collagens and fibronectin

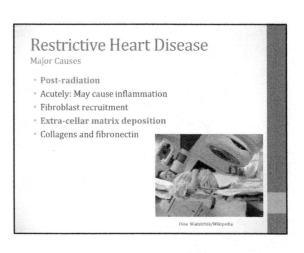

Restrictive Heart Disease
Major Causes

- Pericarditis may occur acutely after therapy
- Long term effects
  - Pericardial disease
  - Coronary artery disease
  - Valvular disease
  - Conduction abnormalities
- Restrictive cardiomyopathy
  - Fibrous tissue accumulation
  - Diastolic dysfunction

Restrictive Heart Disease
Major Causes

- Loeffler's syndrome
  - Hypereosinophilic syndrome
  - High eosinophil count
  - Eosinophilic infiltration of organs
- Skin (eczema)
- Lungs (fibrosis)

Bobjgalindo/Wikipedia

Restrictive Heart Disease
Major Causes

- Primary HES
  - Neoplastic disorder
  - Stem cell, myeloid, or eosinophilic neoplasm
- Secondary HES
  - Reactive process
  - Eosinophilic overproduction due to cytokines
  - Occurs in parasitic infections (ascaris lumbricoides)
  - Some tumors/lymphomas
- Idiopathic HES

Bobjgalindo/Wikipedia

Restrictive Heart Disease
Major Causes

- Eosinophilic infiltration of myocardium
  - Common mode of death
- Acute phase
  - Myocarditis (often asymptomatic)
- Chronic phase
  - Endomyocardial fibrosis and myocyte death
  - Can see restrictive heart disease
  - Thrombus formation common (embolic stroke)

Bobjgalindo/Wikipedia

Restrictive Heart Disease
Major Causes

- Endocardial fibroelastosis
  - Endocardial thickening (innermost myocardium)
  - Infants in first year of life
  - Thick myocardium
  - Proliferation of fibrous (collagen) and elastic fibers
- Restrictive cardiomyopathy

Avsar Aras

Acute Heart Failure

Jason Ryan, MD, MPH

Heart Failure
Acute vs. Chronic — **Fluid overload**

Acute	Chronic
Congested/Swollen	Euvolemic
Pulmonary Edema	Clear lungs
Pitting Edema	No pitting edema
↑JVP	JVP flat

Acute Exacerbations
Causes

- #1: Dietary indiscretion
  - High salt intake
- #2: Poor medication compliance

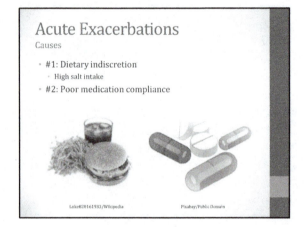

LukeH20161933/Wikipedia   Pixabay/Public Domain

Dietary Indiscretion

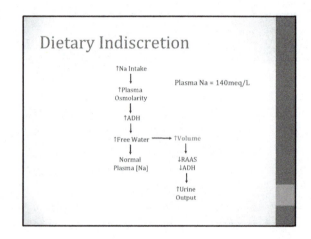

Plasma Na = 140meq/L

Acute Exacerbations
Causes

- Infection/trauma/surgery
  - Activation of sympathetic nervous system
- Ischemia (rare)
  - Decreased cardiac output
- **NSAIDs**
  - Inhibit cyclooxygenase (COX) → ↓ prostaglandins
  - Prostaglandins maintain renal perfusion
  - Result: Less renal perfusion → salt/water retention

Acute Heart Failure Therapy

- Often treated in the hospital
- Goal: Symptom relief
  - Contrast with chronic HF: reduce mortality/hospitalizations
- Often same therapies for diastolic versus systolic

Loop Diuretics

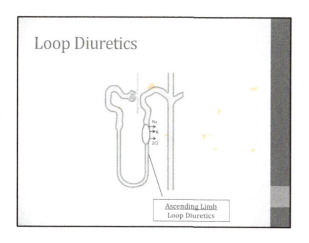

Ascending Limb
Loop Diuretics

Loop Diuretics
Furosemide, Bumetanide, Torsemide, Ethacrynic Acid

- Inhibit Na-K-Cl pump in ascending loop of Henle
- Result in salt-water excretion
- Relieve congestion
- IV better than PO (gut is swollen) — *IV is better*
- Key side effects
    - Hypokalemia
    - Volume depletion (Renal failure; hypotension)
- Sulfonamide drugs: allergy (except ethacrynic acid)

Metolazone

- Thiazide-like diuretic
- Inhibits Na-Cl reabsorption distal tubule
- Gives loop diuretics a "kick"
- Vigorous diuresis
- Side effects: additional fluid, K+ loss

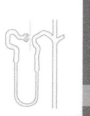

Nitrates

- Predominant mechanism is venous dilation
    - Bigger veins hold more blood
    - Takes blood away from left ventricle
    - Lowers LVEDV (preload), LA pressure
    - Less pulmonary edema → improved dyspnea

Nitrates

- Side effects
    - Headache (meningeal vasodilation)
    - Flushing
    - Hypotension

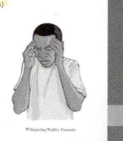

Wikipedia/Public Domain

Vasodilators
"Afterload reduction"

- ACE inhibitors
- Hydralazine
- Cause peripheral vasodilation
- Reduced afterload → increased cardiac output

Nitrates plus Hydralazine

- **Combination therapy for acute and chronic HF**
  - Studied in systolic heart failure
  - Reduction in preload (nitrates) and afterload (hydralazine)
  - Acute therapy: Improves symptoms
  - Chronic therapy: Lowers mortality in some studies
- Largely replaced by ACE inhibitors
- Some studies suggested benefit in **black patients**

Inotropes

- Increase contractility
- Only for **systolic heart failure**
  - No role in diastolic heart failure (normal contractility)
- All activate **β1 pathways in myocytes**
  - Increased HR and contractility
- Can also active **β2 pathways in smooth muscle**
  - Vasodilation → hypotension

Inotropes
Milrinone

- **Phosphodiesterase 3 inhibitor**
  - PD3 breaks down cAMP in myocytes
  - Inhibition → ↑cAMP → contraction
  - Vascular smooth muscle ↑cAMP (β2) → dilation
- ↑Inotropy
- ↑Vasodilation
- Hypotension

Inotropes
Dobutamine

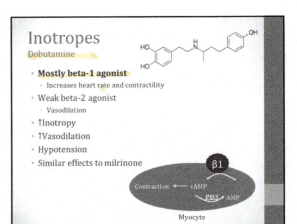

- **Mostly beta-1 agonist**
  - Increases heart rate and contractility
- Weak beta-2 agonist
  - Vasodilation
- ↑Inotropy
- ↑Vasodilation
- Hypotension
- Similar effects to milrinone

Inotropes
Dopamine

- **Does not cross blood brain barrier** (no CNS effects)
- Peripheral effects highly dependent on dose
- <u>Low dose</u>: dopamine agonist
  - Vasodilation in kidneys
- <u>Medium dose</u>: beta-1 agonist
  - Increased heart rate and contractility
- <u>High dose</u>: alpha agonist
  - Vasoconstriction

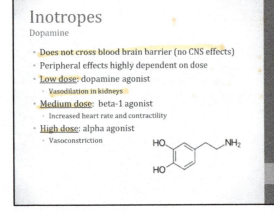

Inotropes
Epinephrine

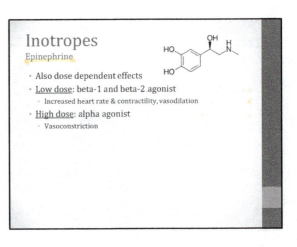

- Also dose dependent effects
- <u>Low dose</u>: beta-1 and beta-2 agonist
  - Increased heart rate & contractility, vasodilation
- <u>High dose</u>: alpha agonist
  - Vasoconstriction

Inotrope Risks

- Numerous registries and clinical trials demonstrate increased mortality with routine use of inotropes
- **Dangerous drugs** used in very sick patients under monitored conditions

A Typical Acute Heart Failure Course

- ER presentation:
  - Dyspnea, edema, sleeping in chair
- Admitted to hospital
  - Nitro drip to relieve dyspnea
  - IV Furosemide to remove fluid
- Hospital Day 2
  - Weight down 4kg, feels better
  - Nitro drip stopped
  - Changed to oral furosemide
- Hospital Day 3: Discharge

A More Complex Heart Failure Course

- ER presentation:
  - Dyspnea, edema, sleeping in chair
  - Known LVEF 10%
- Admitted to hospital
  - Nitro drip to relieve dyspnea
  - IV Furosemide to remove fluid
- Hospital Day 2
  - Poor urine output, Cool extremities, Cr rises 1.1→1.4
  - Dobutamine drip started

A More Complex Heart Failure Course

- Hospital Day 3-5
  - Good urine output
  - Weight loss 4kg
  - Breathing improves
- Hospital Day 6
  - Dobutamine stopped
  - Furosemide drip stopped
- Hospital Day 7
  - Oral furosemide given
- Hospital Day 8: Discharge

Heart Failure Readmission

- Recurrence of HF after discharge common
  - Post-discharge follow-up VERY important
  - "Readmissions" a focus of public health policy
  - High risk of readmission within 30 days
  - Highest risk category among Medicare population

Acute Heart Failure

- Most patients require chronic, daily diuretic
  - Helps to maintain euvolemic status
  - Often oral furosemide or other loop diuretic
- Some patients require daily long acting nitrate
  - Often oral isosorbide mononitrate

Acute Heart Failure

- Rare patients: **continued** treatment for **low output**
  - Systolic heart failure only
  - Chronic, IV infusion inotrope (i.e. "home dobutamine")
  - Left ventricular assist device (LVAD)
  - Heart transplant

Digoxin — only oral

- Only available *oral* inotrope
- "Dig and diuretic" once the mainstay of HF treatment
- What changed?
  - Digoxin shown to have no mortality benefit
  - Digoxin not effective for diastolic heart failure
    - About 50% of all cases
  - Digoxin carries significant risk of side effects

Digoxin Mechanism
Two important cardiac effects

- #1: **Inhibits Na-K-ATPase pump**
  - More Na in cell → more Ca++ in cell
  - More Ca++ → more contractility
- #2 Suppresses AV node conduction (parasympathetic)
  - Can be used to slow heart rate in rapid atrial fibrillation

Digoxin
Benefits in Heart Failure

- Useful for **systolic HF** patients
  - Symptoms despite maximal therapy on other drugs
  - i.e. persistent dyspnea despite good volume status
- Can be administered for acute heart failure
- Can be administered long term to maintain CO

Digoxin
Benefits in Heart Failure

- Increased cardiac output
- Improved symptoms and quality of life
- No established mortality benefit

Chronic Heart Failure

Jason Ryan, MD, MPH

Heart Failure Treatment Pathway

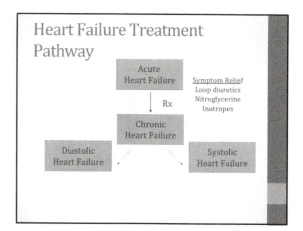

Symptom Relief
Loop diuretics
Nitroglycerine
Inotropes

Chronic Heart Failure

- LOTS of therapies for systolic heart failure
  - Drugs: ACE-inhibitors, beta blockers, aldosterone antagonists
  - Defibrillators
  - Bi-ventricular pacemakers
- NO direct therapies for diastolic heart failure
  - Guidelines recommendations: treat HTN, diabetes, A. fib
  - Mainstay of therapy: monitor for symptoms, diuretics

Systolic Heart Failure

- Chronic over-activation of two physiologic systems
- **Renin-angiotensin-aldosterone system**
- **Sympathetic nervous system (β1 stimulation)**
- Blockade → ↓ mortality and disease progression

Renin-Angiotensin System

Angiotensinogen
+ Renin
AI →+ACE→ A2

ARBs
Sympathetic System
Renal Na/Cl resorption
Arteriolar vasoconstriction
ACE Inhibitors
Adrenal aldosterone secretion
Pituitary ADH secretion

Net Result
↑Salt/Water Retention
↑Preload
↑TPR
↑Afterload

RAAS Drugs

- **ACE Inhibitors**
  - Captopril, Enalapril, Lisinopril, Ramipril
  - Block conversion AI → AII
- **Angiotensin Receptor Blockers (ARBs)**
  - Candesartan, Irbesartan, Valsartan
  - Directly block AII receptor
- Both classes: ↓ morality, ↓hospitalizations
- Side effects
  - Hyperkalemia (↓aldosterone)
  - Renal failure (↓GFR)

ACE Inhibitors
Unique Side Effects

- Due to increased bradykinin
- Dry Cough
  - Occurs in ~10% of patients
- Angioedema
  - Swelling of face, tongue
  - Can be life-threatening

Bradykinin

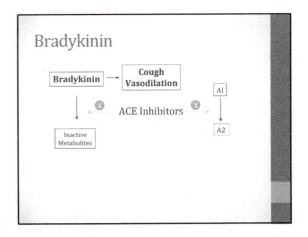

Beta Blockers

- Once contraindicated in systolic heart failure
  - Negative inotropes
- Not used in acute heart failure
  - May worsen cardiac output and symptoms

Beta Blockers

- Three agents beneficial in chronic systolic HF failure
  - Metoprolol (β1)
  - Carvedilol (β1β2α1)
  - Bisoproplol (β1)
- ↓ morality, ↓ hospitalizations

Aldosterone Antagonists

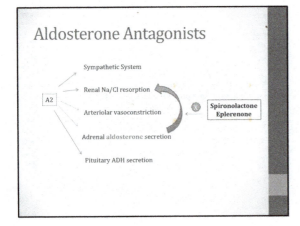

Spironolactone, Eplerenone
Potassium-sparing diuretics

- ↑Na/H₂O excretion (diuretics)
- "Spare" potassium
  - Unlike other diuretics, do not increase K⁺ excretion
- HYPERkalemia is side effect
- Reduced mortality
- Reduced hospitalization rate

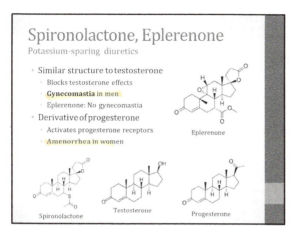

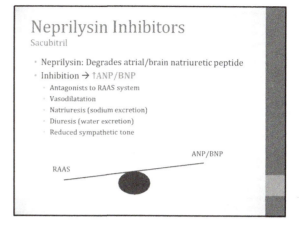

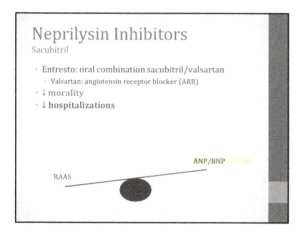

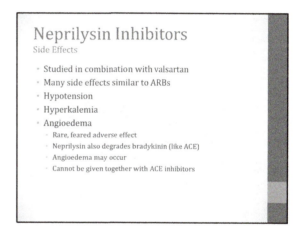

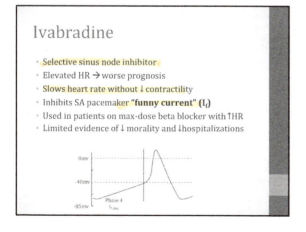

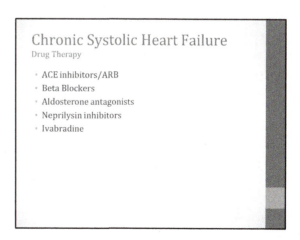

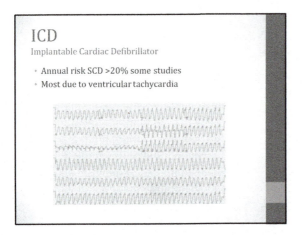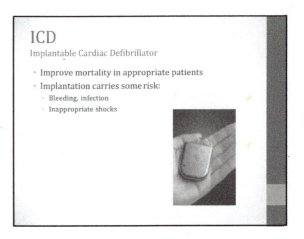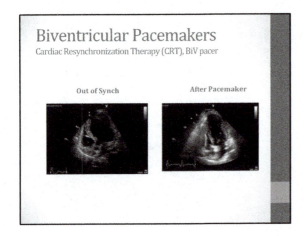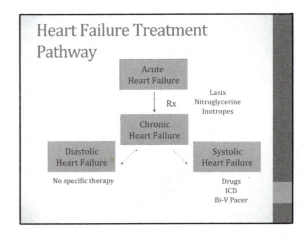

Cardiac Embryology

Jason Ryan, MD, MPH

Primitive Heart
22 days

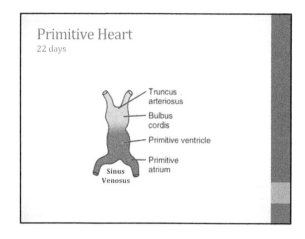

Primitive Heart
22 days

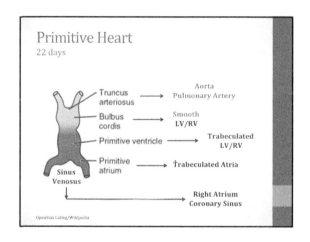

Sinus Venosus

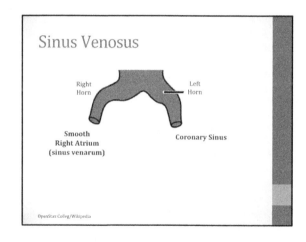

Cardinal Veins

- Form SVC/IVC (not from heart tube)
- Connect to right atrium
- Superior vena cava
  - R common cardinal vein and R anterior cardinal vein
- Inferior vena cava
  - Posterior veins

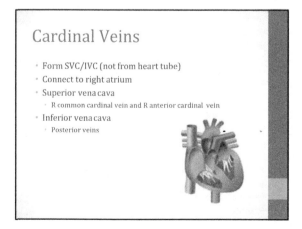

Adult Heart

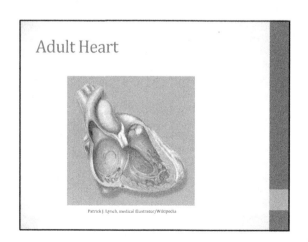

Patrick J. Lynch, medical illustrator/Wikipedia

Primitive Heart

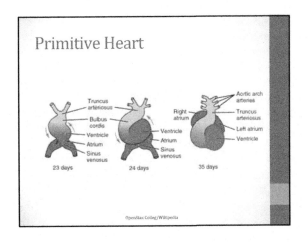

Cardiac Looping

- Heart tube "loops" at about 4 weeks gestation
- Establishes left-right orientation in chest
- Requires cilia and **dynein**
- Dextrocardia (heart on the right side of body)
  - Seen in in Kartagener syndrome
  - Part of primary ciliary dyskinesia

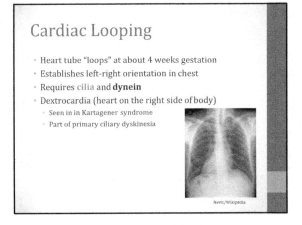

Ventricular Septum Formation

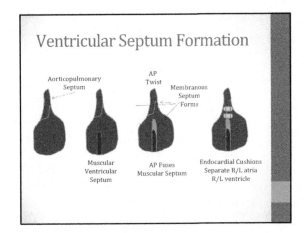

Ventricular Septum Pathology

- Membranous VSD (most common type)
- Muscular VSD

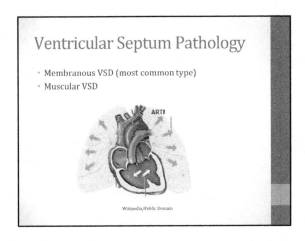

Endocardial Cushions

- Contribute to several cardiac structures
  - Atrial septum
  - Ventricular septum
  - AV valves (mitral/tricuspid)
  - Semilunar valves (aortic/pulmonic)
- **Endocardial cushion defects**
  - Atrioventricular canal defects
  - Atrioventricular septal defects
  - ASD, VSD, Valvular malformations
  - Common in **Down syndrome**

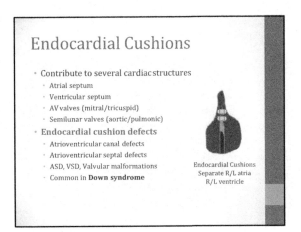

Aorticopulmonary septum
Spiral Septum

- Formed from neural crest cells
- Migrate to truncal and bulbar ridges
- Separates aorta and pulmonary arteries
- Fuses with interventricular septum

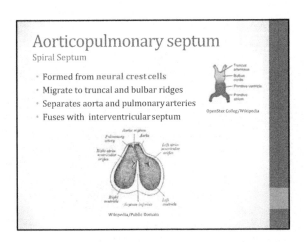

Aorticopulmonary septum
Spiral Septum

- Abnormal formation → congenital pathology
- Transposition of great vessels
  - Failure to spiral
- Tetralogy of Fallot
  - Skewed septum development
- Persistent truncus arteriosus
  - Partial/incomplete septum development

Atrial Septum

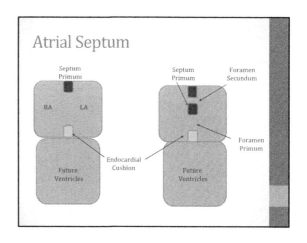

Atrial Septum

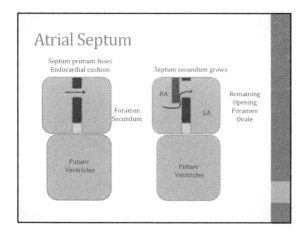

PFO
Patent Foramen Ovale

- Found in ~25% adults
- Failure of foramen ovale to close after birth
- Septum primum/secundum fail to fuse

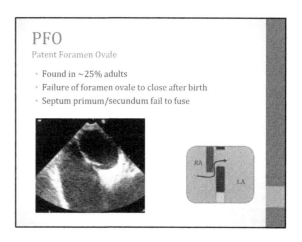

Fetal Circulation

- **High resistance to flow** in lungs
- Oxygenated blood umbilical veins
  - About 80% saturated (30mmHg O2)
- Travels directly to right atrium
  - Bypasses liver via ductus venosus
- Bypasses lungs via foramen ovale
- Some blood gets to RV (SVC)
  - Bypasses lungs via ductus arteriosus
  - Left pulmonary artery to aorta

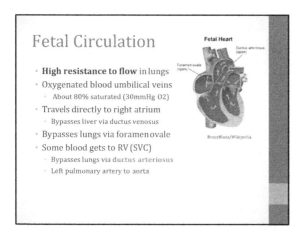

Changes at Birth

- Pulmonary resistance falls
- More blood to left atrium
- LA pressure > RA pressure
- Foramen ovale closes (fossa ovalis)
- Ductus arteriosus closes
  - In utero: ↓ O2, ↑ prostaglandins maintain patency
  - Birth: ↑ O2, ↓ prostaglandins (loss of placenta)

	PVR	RA	LA
In Utero	↑	↑	↓
Birth	↓	↓	↑

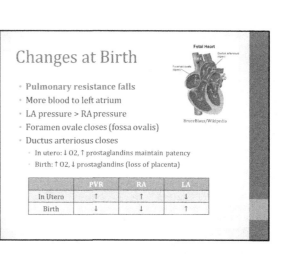

Changes at Birth

- Placenta has low resistance to flow
- In utero: helps keep LA pressure low
- At birth: **increase in peripheral resistance**
- Rise in systemic blood pressure
- Rise in left ventricular pressure
- Contributes to rise in LA pressure

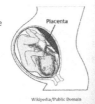

Wikipedia/Public Domain

Shunts

Jason Ryan, MD, MPH

Shunts

RA	LA
RV	LV
PA	Ao

Shunts

- Left side pressures >> Right side pressures
  - LA ~10mmHg >> RA ~6mmHg
  - LV ~120/10 >> RV ~24/6
  - Ao ~ 120/80 >> PA ~24/12
- Left to right connection → Left to right flow
  - VSD (LV→RV)
  - ASD (LA→RA)
  - PDA (Aorta → Left pulm artery)

Shunts

- At birth:
  - Left to right flow → volume overload of right heart
  - Blood flow to lungs unimpaired → no cyanosis
- YEARS later (untreated)
  - Pulmonary vessels become stiff/thick
  - Right ventricle hypertrophies
  - Right sided pressures rise
  - Shunt reverses (now R → L)
  - Cyanosis occurs (Eisenmenger syndrome)
- "Blue kids" not "blue babies"

VSD
Ventricular Septal Defect

- Most common congenital anomaly
- Communication LV/RV
- Harsh, holosystolic murmur
  - Tricuspid area (LLSB)

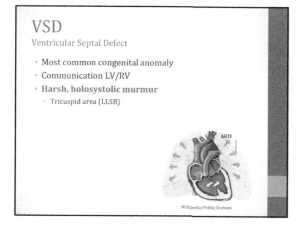

Wikipedia/Public Domain

VSD
Ventricular Septal Defect

- Characterized in many ways
  - Size
  - Location
  - Associated defects

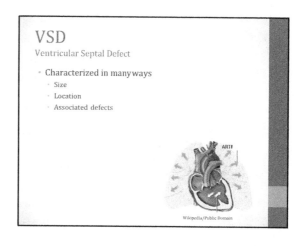

Wikipedia/Public Domain

VSD
Ventricular Septal Defect

- Small VSD
  - Tiny hole → resists flow across defect ("restrictive")
  - Lots of turbulence → loud murmur
  - Small shunt (small volume of flow across defect)
- Large VSD
  - Large hole ("non-restrictive")
  - Significant shunting
  - Often closed surgically

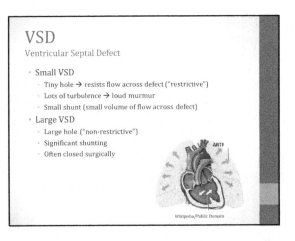

Wikipedia/Public Domain

ASD
Atrial Septal Defect

- Communication between left/right atrium
- Adds volume to RA/RV
- Delays closure of pulmonic valve
- **Wide, fixed splitting of S2**
- Increased flow across PV/TV
- **Systolic ejection murmur**
- Rarely a mid-diastolic murmur

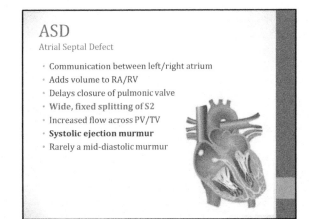

ASD
Atrial Septal Defect

- Oxygenated blood LA → RA
- ↑ O2 saturation in RA, RV, PA
- "Shunt run"
  - Series of blood samples
  - SVC = 65%
  - IVC = 65%
  - RA = 75%
  - RV = 75% — "Step up"
  - PA = 75%

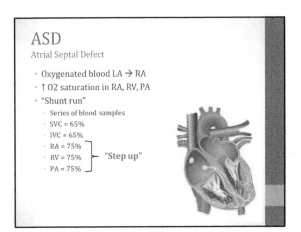

ASD
Atrial Septal Defect

- **Secundum type is most common**
  - Defects at site of foramen ovale/ostium secundum
  - Poor growth of secundum septum
  - Or excessive absorption of primum septum
  - Located mid-septum
  - Often isolated defect

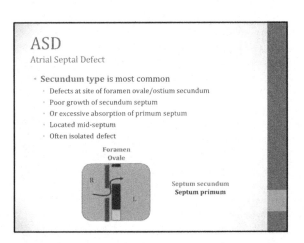

Septum secundum
Septum primum

ASD
Atrial Septal Defect

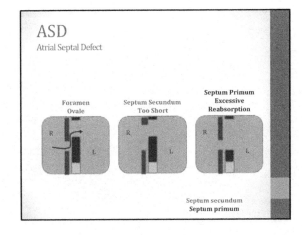

Septum secundum
Septum primum

ASD
Atrial Septal Defect

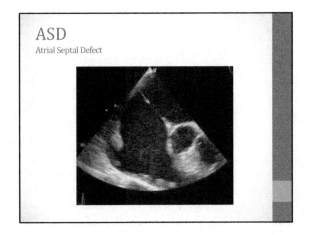

ASD
Atrial Septal Defect

- Primum type
  - Defect at site of ostium primum
  - Failure of primum septum to fuse with endocardial cushions
  - Located near AV valves; often occurs with other defects
  - Seen in endocardial cushion defects (Down syndrome)

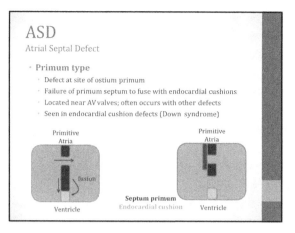

ASD
Atrial Septal Defect

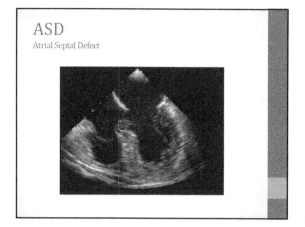

PDA
Patent Ductus Arteriosus

- Ductus arteriosus shunts blood in utero
  - Left pulmonary artery → aorta
- Closes close after birth
  - "Functional" closure 18 to 24 hours (smooth muscle)
  - "Anatomic" occlusion over next few days/weeks
  - Becomes **ligamentum arteriosum**
- Patency maintained by prostaglandin E2
  - Major source in utero is placenta

PDA
Patent Ductus Arteriosus

- Rarely remains patent (3 to 8 per 10,000 births)
- Associated with congenital rubella syndrome
  - ToRCHeS infection
  - Mother: Rash, fever, lymphadenopathy
  - Baby: Deafness, cataracts, cardiac disease
  - PDA common
  - Rare in developed countries (vaccination)
  - Consider in infants whose mothers are immigrants

PDA
Patent Ductus Arteriosus

- **Continuous, machine-like murmur**
- **Widened pulse pressure**
  - Loss of volume in arterial tree through PDA
  - Low diastolic pressure → Increased pulse pressure
- **Differential cyanosis**
  - Occurs when shunt reverses R → L
  - Blue toes, normal fingers

Alprostadil

- Prostaglandin E1
- Maintains patency of ductus arteriosus
- Key effect: delivers blood to lungs
- Useful when poor RV → PA blood flow
  - Tetralogy of Fallot
  - Pulmonary atresia

Indomethacin

- NSAID
- Inhibits cyclooxygenase
- Decreases prostaglandin formation
- Can be used to close PDA

Qp:Qs

- Qp = Pulmonary blood flow
- Qs = Systemic blood flow
- Qp:Qs should be 1:1
- In shunts, Qp:Qs may be > 1:1
  - 1.5:1, 2:1, 3:1, etc.

Eisenmenger's Syndrome

- Uncorrected ASD/VSD/PDA
- Right heart chronically overloaded
  - RV Hypertrophy
  - Pulmonary hypertension
- Shunt reverses right → left
  - Cyanosis
  - Clubbing
  - Polycythemia (very high Hct)

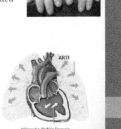

Wikipedia/Public Domain

Fetal Alcohol Syndrome

- Caused by prenatal exposure to alcohol (teratogen)
- Characteristic facial features
- Impaired neurologic function
- Congenital heart defects
  - Atrial septal defect
  - Ventricular septal defect
  - Tetralogy of Fallot

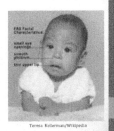

Teresa Kellerman/Wikipedia

PFO
Patent Foramen Ovale

- Found in ~25% adults
- Failure of foramen ovale to close after birth
- Can lead to **stroke** in patients with DVT/PE

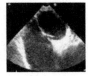

Cyanotic Congenital Heart Disease

Jason Ryan, MD, MPH

Cyanosis

- **Central** cyanosis
  - Cardiac output normal
  - Blood is flowing
  - Not enough O2
  - Lips
  - Nail beds
  - Conjunctivae
  - Warm extremities
- Peripheral cyanosis
  - Low blood flow
  - Severe heart failure
  - Cold extremities

WaltFletcher/Wikipedia

Blue Babies

- Central cyanosis early in life
- Blood not going through lungs after birth
  - Tetralogy of Fallot
  - Transposition of great vessels
  - Truncus arteriosus
  - Tricuspid atresia
  - Total anomalous pulmonary venous return

Tetralogy of Fallot

- Constellation of four abnormalities
  - Ventricular septal defect (VSD)
  - Rightward deviation of aortic valve ("overriding aorta")
  - Subpulmonary stenosis
  - Right ventricular hypertrophy

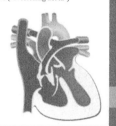

Infundibulum
Conus Arteriosus

- "Funnel" leading to pulmonic valve
- Develops from bulbus cordis
- Smooth, muscular structure at RV outflow to PA

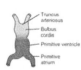

OpenStax College/Wikipedia

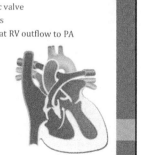

Infundibulum
Conus Arteriosus

- **Septum displaced (moves toward RV) in TOF**
- Causes "overriding aorta"
  - 5-95% of aorta may lie over RV
- Causes VSD
  - Usually large ("non-restrictive")

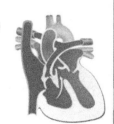

Infundibulum
Conus Arteriosus

- "Infundibular stenosis"
  - Subpulmonary stenosis
  - RV outflow tract obstruction
- Abnormal pulmonary valve
  - Rarely main cause of obstruction
- Flow obstruction → RVH

Tetralogy of Fallot
Physiology

- High resistance to flow RV → pulmonary artery
  - RV outflow pulmonic stenosis
- Diverts blood across VSD to left ventricle
- **Severity of flow obstruction determines symptoms**
- Severe obstruction: severe cyanosis
- Mild obstruction: less shunting ("pink" tets)

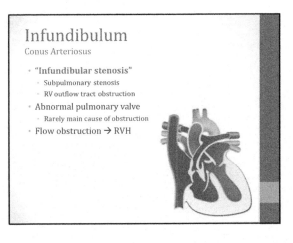

Tetralogy of Fallot
Physiology

- Poor blood flow RV → lungs
- Left to right shunts beneficial
  - Bring back to pulmonary artery
  - Diverts blood to lungs
  - Improves oxygenation
  - **Patent ductus arteriosus**
  - Aortopulmonary collateral arteries
  - Surgical shunt

Tetralogy of Fallot
Murmur

- Systolic ejection murmur
  - Crescendo-decrescendo
  - RV outflow and pulmonic stenosis
  - Heard best at left sternal border
- Single S2
  - S2 = closure of aortic and pulmonic valves
  - TOF: Diseased pulmonic valve → no sound
- VSD murmur (holosystolic) not typically heard
  - Large VSD → no murmur

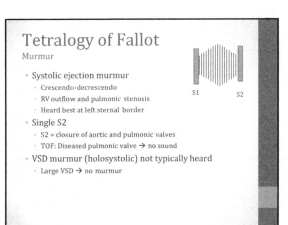

S1   S2

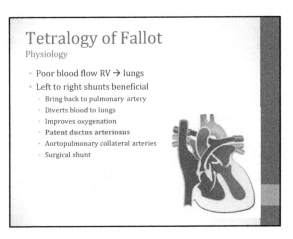

Tetralogy of Fallot
X-ray

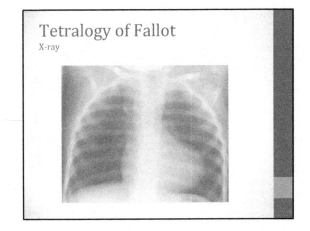

Tetralogy of Fallot
Other Features

- **Squatting improves symptoms**
  - Increased afterload/TPR (resists flow out of LV)
  - Pressure rises in the aorta/left ventricle
  - Less blood shunted RV → LV via VSD
  - More blood to lungs

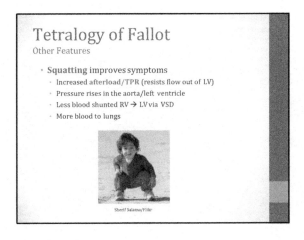

Sherif Salama/Flikr

Tetralogy of Fallot
Other Features

- **"Tet spells"**
  - Sudden cyanosis often when agitated
  - Severe/complete RVOT obstruction
  - O2, knees to chest, beta blockers (propranolol)

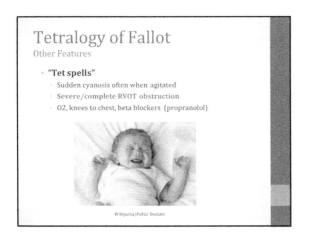

Truncus Arteriosus

- Common arterial trunk → Mixing of blood
- Failure of **neural crest cells** to drive formation of aorticopulmonary septum
- Almost always has VSD

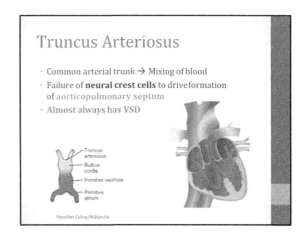

Transposition of Great Vessels

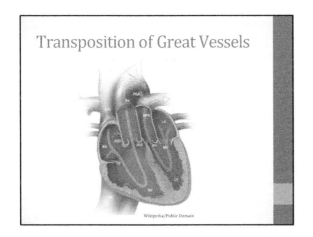

Transposition of Great Vessels

- Normal heart:
  - Aorta is posterior and to right of pulmonary artery

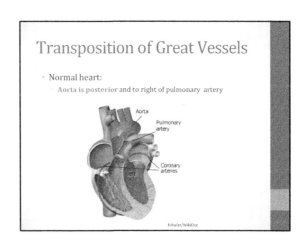

Transposition of Great Vessels

- D-transposition (most common type):
  - Aorta forms anterior and rightward of pulmonary artery
  - Aorta arises from right ventricle
  - Pulmonary artery from left ventricle

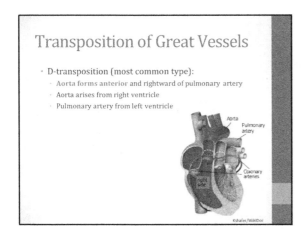

Transposition of Great Vessels

- RV → Aorta → body → RA → RV
- LV → Pulmonary artery → LA → LV
- Two completely separate circuits
- NOT compatible with life unless shunt present
  - Usually PDA or VSD

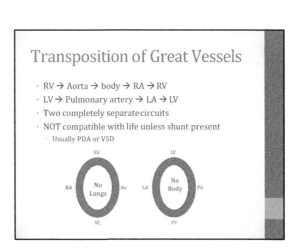

L-TGA
L-Transposition of the Great Arteries

- "Double switch": Aorta/PA and LA/RA
- "Congenitally corrected TGA"
- Venous blood → RA → LV → PA → Lungs
- Lungs → PV → LA → RV → Aorta
- Two circuits *not* separated
- Wrong connections (RV-Aorta, LV-PA)
- **Eventually right ventricle fails**

Maternal Diabetes

- Infants at increased risk congenital anomalies
- Common congenital heart defects
  - Transposition of great vessels
  - Truncus arteriosus
  - Tricuspid atresia
  - VSD
  - PDA

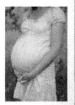

Tricuspid Atresia

- Abnormal AV valves from endocardial cushions
- **No tricuspid valve**
- No blood RA → RV

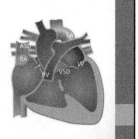

Tricuspid Atresia

- All cases have R→L shunt
  - Always seen with ASD
  - Allows blood flow to LA
- All cases have L→R shunt
  - Allows blood flow to lungs
  - LV → RV via VSD
  - Ao → PA via PDA

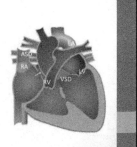

TAPVR
Total Anomalous Pulmonary Venous Return

- Normal: pulmonary veins drain to left atrium
- TAPVR: pulmonary veins drain to venous system
  - Innominate (brachiocephalic) veins → SVC
  - Coronary sinus
  - Portal vein

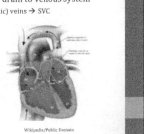

TAPVR
Total Anomalous Pulmonary Venous Return

- RV → Lungs → Pulm Veins → RA → RV
- RA and RV dilate
- Must have a right to left shunt
  - ASD (most common)
  - PDA
- Mixed (low O2) blood to body

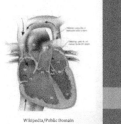

Ebstein's Anomaly

- Apical displacement of TV → small RV
- "Atrialization" of RV tissue
- Severe tricuspid regurgitation
- Can lead to right heart failure

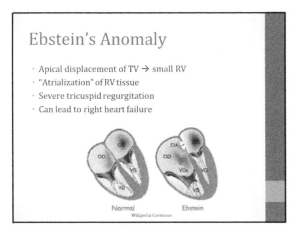

Ebstein's Anomaly

- Right to left shunting and cyanosis if ASD
  - High RA pressure
- Associated with **WPW**
  - Electrical bypass tract often present
  - Delta wave on EKG

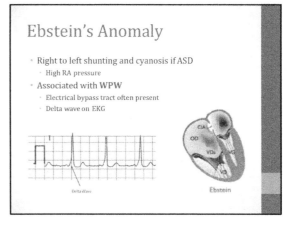

Maternal Lithium

- Teratogen
- Completely equilibrates across the placenta
- Teratogenic effects primarily involve heart
- **Ebstein's anomaly** most common

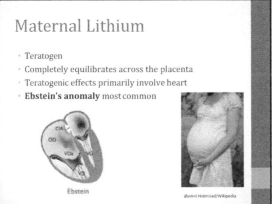
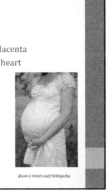

Pulmonary Atresia

- Failure of pulmonic valve orifice to develop
- No flow from RV to lungs
- In utero blood bypasses lungs (normal development)
- At birth: No blood flow to lungs through PV
  - PVR should fall but does not
- Often co-exists with VSD for outflow of RV
  - Similar to a severe form of Tetralogy of Fallot
- Survival depends on ductus arteriosus
- Alprostadil given to keep DA open

Pulmonary Atresia

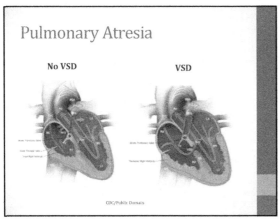

Alprostadil

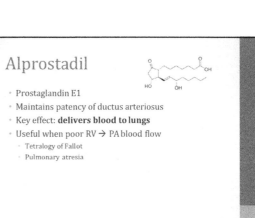

- Prostaglandin E1
- Maintains patency of ductus arteriosus
- Key effect: **delivers blood to lungs**
- Useful when poor RV → PA blood flow
  - Tetralogy of Fallot
  - Pulmonary atresia

Conotruncal Heart Defects

- Outflow tract anomalies
  - Trunk = Truncus arteriosus
  - Conus = Conus arteriosus
- Tetralogy of Fallot
- Truncus arteriosus
- Transposition of the great arteries
- **22q deletion syndromes**
  - DiGeorge syndrome (Thymic Aplasia)
  - Immunodeficiency, hypocalcemia
  - Conotruncal anomalies

Coarctation of the Aorta

Jason Ryan, MD, MPH

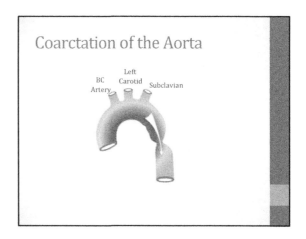

Coarctation of the Aorta

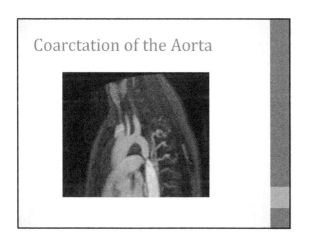

Coarctation of the Aorta

- Congenital disorder
- Usually involves thoracic aorta distal to subclavian
- Near insertion of ductus arteriosus
- "Juxtaductal" aorta
- Subtypes based on location of ductus arteriosus
- High **resistance to flow** in aorta

Coarctation of the Aorta

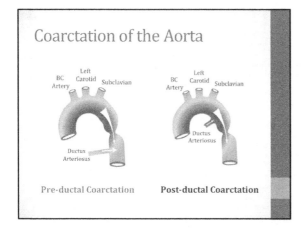

Pre-ductal Coarctation   **Post-ductal Coarctation**

Ductus Arteriosus

- Shunts blood in utero
- Left pulmonary artery → aorta
- Patency maintained by ↓O2 and ↑ prostaglandins
- At birth: ↑O2 and ↓ prostaglandins
- "Functional" closure 18 to 24 hours after birth
  - Smooth muscle constriction
- "Anatomic" occlusion over next few days/weeks
- Becomes **ligamentum arteriosum**

Coarctation of the Aorta
Preductal or Infantile

- Ductus arteriosus supplies lower extremities
- Poor development of collateral vessels

Coarctation of the Aorta
Preductal or Infantile

- At birth ductus arteriosus open (not closed yet)
- Deoxygenated blood to lower extremity
- Lower extremity cyanosis may occur

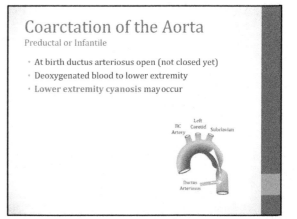

Coarctation of the Aorta
Preductal or Infantile

- Ductus closure → symptoms may develop
- All flow through aorta with severe narrowing
- Abrupt increase afterload
- Rise in LVEDP
- Acute heart failure
- LV can dilate → fail → shock
- All caused by **closure of DA**

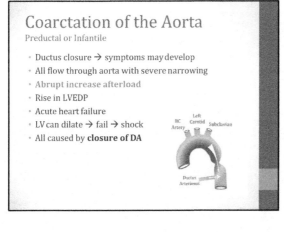

Coarctation of the Aorta
Preductal or Infantile

- Key associations: Turner syndrome (45, XO)
- Short stature, webbed neck
- 5-10% have coarctation of the aorta

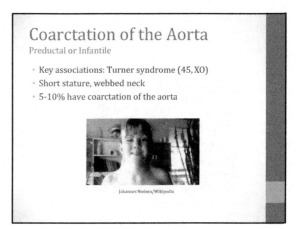

Coarctation of the Aorta
Postductal or Adult type

- Ductus arteriosus does not supply lower extremities
- Collaterals develop
- May go undetected until adulthood

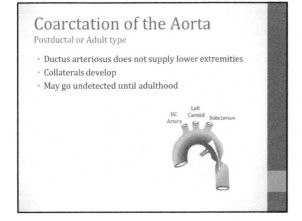

Coarctation of the Aorta

- Lower extremities → low blood pressure
  - ↑ Renin release
  - Salt/water retention
  - Vasoconstriction (AII)
  - Weak pulses ("brachio-femoral delay")
- Upper extremities and head → **high blood pressure**
- Secondary hypertension

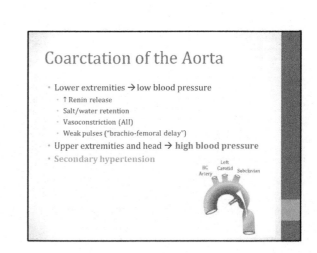

Coarctation of the Aorta

- Key association: **bicuspid aortic valve**
- Found in up to 60% of coarctation cases

Patrick J. Lynch, medical illustrator

Coarctation of the Aorta

- Key association: **intracranial aneurysms**
- Occur in about 10% of patients with coarctation

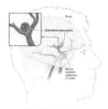

Wikipedia/Public Domain

Coarctation of the Aorta
Signs/Symptoms

- Only sign may be hypertension in arms
- Murmur over back between scapula
- Weak femoral pulses
- Pain with walking (claudication)

Coarctation of the Aorta
Signs/Symptoms

- **Rib notching**
  - High pressure above coarctation
  - Intercostals enlarge to carry blood around obstruction
  - Bulge into ribs
  - "Rib notching" seen on chest x-ray

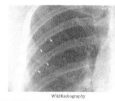

WikiRadiography

Coarctation of the Aorta
Signs/Symptoms

- 3-sign
  - Bulge before and after coarctation
  - "3 sign" on chest x-ray

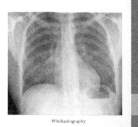

WikiRadiography

Coarctation of the Aorta
Physiology

- **Autoregulation** maintains regional blood flow
  - Normal upper/lower perfusion despite high/low pressures
- Upper extremities
  - High blood pressure → high flow
  - Arterioles constrict to limit flow to normal level
  - Local effect – not mediated by sympathetic/parasympathetic
  - Resistance to flow is high ($Q = \Delta P / R$)
- Lower extremities
  - Low blood pressure
  - Arterioles dilate to increase flow to normal level ($Q = \Delta P / R$)
- Result is normal ("compensated") flow

Coarctation of the Aorta
Complications

- Heart failure
  - Pressure overload of left ventricle
- Aortic rupture/dissection
- **Endocarditis/endarteritis**
  - High-low pressure across narrowing
  - Endothelial injury
  - Low pressure distal to narrowing
  - Bacteria may attach more easily

Hypertension

Jason Ryan, MD, MPH

Hypertension
- Blood pressure >140/90
- Need more than one measurement

Etiology
- Most (90%) is primary ("essential") HTN
  - Cause not clear
- Remainder (10%) secondary

Hypertension
Risk Factors
- Family history
- African-American race
- High salt intake
- Alcohol
- Obesity
- Physical inactivity

Sodium Intake

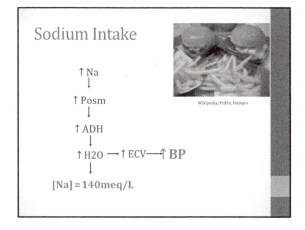

↑ Na
↓
↑ Posm
↓
↑ ADH
↓
↑ H2O → ↑ ECV → ↑ **BP**
↓
[Na] = 140 meq/L

Wikipedia/Public Domain

Hypertension
Associations
- Stroke
- Heart disease
  - MI
  - Heart failure
- Renal failure
- Aortic aneurysm
- Aortic dissection

Hypertension Effects

- Atherosclerosis – lipid/fibrous plaques in vessels
- Arteriosclerosis – thickening of artery wall
  - Response to chronic hypertension

Hypertension Effects

- **Hyaline** arteriosclerosis
  - Thickening of small arteries
  - Seen with aging
  - Also common with diabetes

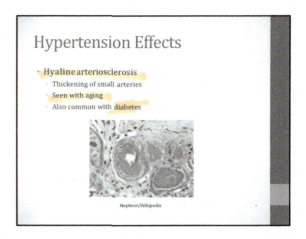

Nephron/Wikipedia

Hypertension Effects

- **Hyperplastic** arteriosclerosis
  - Arteries look like "onion skin"
  - Occurs when hypertension is severe (usually DBP>120)
  - "Malignant" hypertension
  - Retinal hemorrhages, exudates, or papilledema

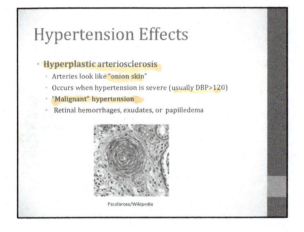

Pacolarosa/Wikipedia

Arteriolar Rarefaction

- Loss of arterioles
- Arterioles close off and get resorbed

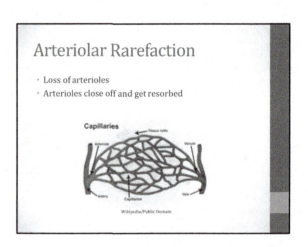

Wikipedia/Public Domain

Hypertension Effects

- **Pulse pressure may increase**
  - Example: Normal 120/80; HTN 170/100
  - Stiff arteries → ↓compliance

$C = \Delta V / \Delta P$

$\Delta P = \Delta V / C$

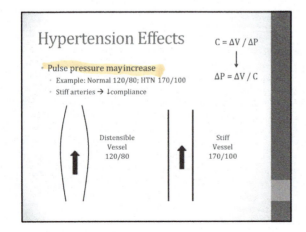

Distensible Vessel 120/80

Stiff Vessel 170/100

Hypertension Effects

- **Afterload on heart is increased**
- Left ventricle: concentric hypertrophy
  - Large voltage on EKG
  - Displaced apical impulse
  - S4

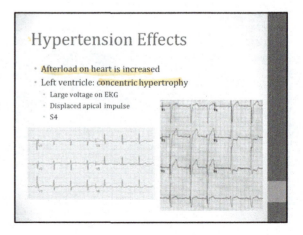

Hypertensive Urgency

- Severe hypertension **without end-organ damage**
- No agreed upon BP value
- **Usually >180/120**

Hypertensive Emergency

- Also no definite value
- **BP usually >180/120** ← Is there is end organ damage
- Patient **longstanding HTN, stops meds**
- Neurologic impairment
  - Retinal hemorrhages, encephalopathy
- Renal impairment
  - Acute renal failure
  - Hematuria, proteinuria
- Cardiac ischemia

Hypertensive Emergency

- Associated with MAHA
- Endothelial injury → thrombus formation
- Improved with BP control

Database Center for Life Science (DBCLS)

Malignant Hypertension

- Historical term
- Most cases **hypertension: "benign"**
  - Modestly elevated blood pressure
  - **Stable over years**
- "Malignant hypertension"
  - Rare form, often fatal
  - Severe elevation of blood pressure (diastolic >120mmHg)
  - Rapidly progressive over 1 to 2 years
  - Renal failure, retinal hemorrhages, ischemia

Secondary Hypertension

Jason Ryan, MD, MPH

Etiology

- Most (90%) is primary ("essential") HTN
  - Cause not clear
- Remainder (10%) secondary

Blood Pressure
Determinants

- Cardiac output
  - Increased with renal salt/water retention
- Total peripheral resistance
  - Key vessels: arterioles
  - Increased by vasoconstrictors (i.e. catecholamines)
  - Increased by sympathetic nervous system

$$BP = CO \times TPR$$

Chronic Kidney Disease

- Over 80% of patients have hypertension
- Multiple causes:
  - Sodium retention
  - Increased renin-angiotensin-aldosterone activity
  - Increased sympathetic nervous system activity

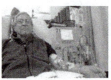

Obstructive Sleep Apnea

- Sleep-related breathing disorder
- Apnea during sleep
- Often associated with hypertension
- Treatment may reduce BP

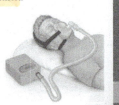

NSAIDs
Ibuprofen, naproxen, indomethacin, ketorolac, diclofenac

- Nonsteroidal anti-inflammatory drugs
- Inhibit cyclooxygenase in kidneys
- Decrease synthesis of prostaglandins
- PGE-2: Renal vasodilator

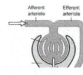

NSAIDs
Ibuprofen, naproxen, indomethacin, ketorolac, diclofenac

- ↓ Na/Water excretion
- May cause hypertension
- May exacerbate heart failure

Vasoconstriction
↓RBF
↓GFR

Oral Contraceptive Pills
OCPs

- Estrogen and progesterone analogs
- Cause mild increase in blood pressure

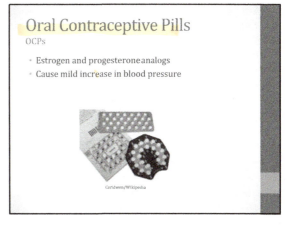

Pseudoephedrine

- Nasal decongestant
- Alpha-1 agonist
- Vasoconstriction → ↓ nasal blood flow

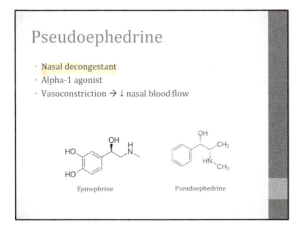

Epinephrine   Pseudoephedrine

Cyclosporine & Tacrolimus

- Immunosuppressants
- Calcineurin inhibitors
- Renal vasoconstriction → salt/water retention
- Diltiazem: drug of choice
  - Impairs metabolism (↑ drug levels)
  - Treats HTN and allows lower dose cyclosporine to be used

Primary Aldosteronism

- Excessive levels of aldosterone secretion
- Not due to increased activity of RAAS system
- Adrenal adenoma (Conn's syndrome)
- Bilateral idiopathic adrenal hyperplasia

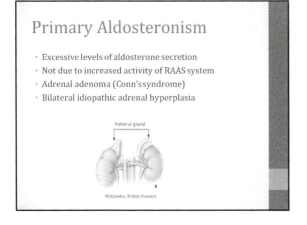

Primary Aldosteronism

- ↑Na reabsorption distal nephron
- ↑ECV → ↑CO → Hypertension
- ↑K excretion → hypokalemia

Aldosterone Escape

- Excess aldosterone does not lead to volume overload
- Usually no pitting edema, rales, increased JVP
- Na/Fluid retention → hypertension
- Compensatory mechanisms activated
  - Increased ANP
- Increased sodium and free water excretion
- Result: diuresis → **normal volume status**

Primary Aldosteronism

- Clinical features
  - Resistant hypertension
  - Hypokalemia
  - Normal volume status on physical exam
- Diagnosis
  - Renin-independent aldosterone section
  - Low plasma renin activity
  - High aldosterone levels
- Drugs of choice: **Spironolactone/Eplerenone**
  - Aldosterone antagonists

Liddle's Syndrome

- Genetic disorder
- **Increased activity of ENaC**
- Similar clinical syndrome to hyperaldosteronism
  - Hypertension
  - Hypokalemia
- **Aldosterone levels low**

Collecting Duct

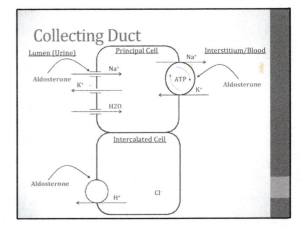

Pheochromocytoma

- **Catecholamine-secreting tumor**
  - Epinephrine, norepinephrine, dopamine
- Usually arises from adrenal gland
- Triad: **Palpitations, headache, episodic sweating**
  - PHEochromocytoma
- Most patient have hypertension
- Diagnosis: Catecholamines breakdown products
  - Metanephrines
  - Vanillylmandelic acid (VMA)

Cushing's Syndrome

- Excess cortisol
- Often from steroid administration
- Other causes
  - Cushing's Disease (pituitary oversecretes ACTH)
  - Tumors (i.e. small cell lung cancer secretes ACTH)
  - Adrenal tumor secretes cortisol
- Cortisol → hypertension
  - Increased vascular sensitivity to adrenergic agonists

Renal Artery Stenosis

- Vascular disease of renal arteries
- Decreased blood flow to kidneys
- Key exam finding: **renal bruit**

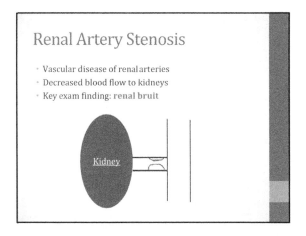

Renal Artery Stenosis

- Increased renin, salt-water retention → HTN
- Often unilateral stenosis
- Normal kidney compensates
- Results: **No signs of volume overload**

Renal Artery Stenosis

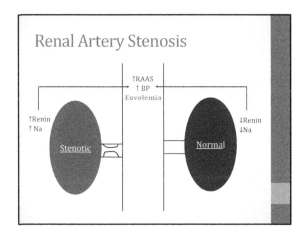

Renal Artery Stenosis
Angiotensin II

- Normal GFR depends on angiotensin II
  - AII → efferent arteriole vasoconstriction
  - Maintains GFR
- ACE inhibitors can precipitate renal failure

Fibromuscular Dysplasia

- Vascular disease → obstruction to flow
- Common among women
- Often occurs in 40s-50s
- Non-atherosclerotic, non-inflammatory
- Often involves medial layer fibroplasia
- Stenosis and aneurysms of vessels ("string of beads")
- Most common in renal and carotid arteries
- Can lead to renal artery stenosis

Coarctation of the Aorta

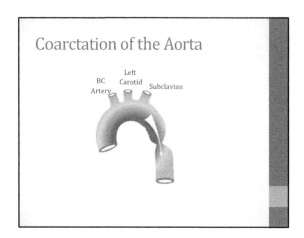

ADPKD
Autosomal dominant polycystic kidney disease

- Genetic disorder
- Mutations of PKD1 or PKD2
- Presents in adulthood with HTN and renal cysts
- Increased RAAS activity

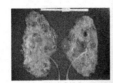
Wikipedia/Public Domain

Antihypertensives

Jason Ryan, MD, MPH

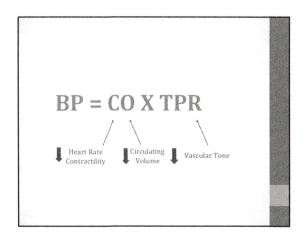

$BP = CO \times TPR$

↓ Heart Rate Contractility ↓ Circulating Volume ↓ Vascular Tone

Beta Receptors

- **β1 receptors in heart, kidneys**
  - Increase heart rate and contractility
  - Stimulate renin release
  - Blockade → ↓ CO, ↓ ECV → ↓ BP
- **β2 receptors**
  - Dilate blood vessels (muscle, liver)
  - Bronchodilate
  - Blockade does not lead to lower blood pressure

Beta Blockers
β1-selective antagonists

- Atenolol, Metoprolol, Esmolol
- Used for hypertension
  - Blockade → ↓ CO, ↓ ECV → ↓ BP
- **Metoprolol: Systolic heart failure**
  - Blocks sympathetic stimulation of heart
  - Reduces mortality

Beta Blockers
β1β2 (nonselective) antagonists

- **Propranolol**, Timolol, Nadolol
- Can be used for hypertension
- Nadolol, Propranolol: Used in **portal hypertension**
  - Beta 1 blockade: ↓ CO, ↓ ECV → ↓ BP
  - Beta 2 blockade: ↓ portal blood flow
- Timolol: Used in **glaucoma**
  - Beta 1 and Beta 2 → aqueous humor production

Beta Blockers
β1β2α1

- Carvedilol, Labetalol
- **Labetalol: Hypertensive Emergency**
  - Rapid reduction in blood pressure
- **Carvedilol: Systolic heart failure**
  - Blocks sympathetic stimulation of heart
  - Reduces mortality

Beta Blockers
Partial Agonists

- Pindolol: β1β2 (nonselective)
- Acebutolol: β1-selective
- "Intrinsic sympathomimetic activity"
  - Beta agonist when sympathetic activity is low
  - Beta blocker when sympathetic activity is high
- Can cause **angina** through beta 1 activation
- Special pharmacologic properties

Beta Blockers
Side effects

- Fatigue, erectile dysfunction, depression
  - More common with older beta blockers (propranolol)
- Hyperlipidemia
  - Mild increase in triglycerides
  - Mild decrease in HDL
  - Effect varies with different beta blockers

Beta Blockers
Side effects

- Caution in diabetes
- Blockade of epinephrine effects
  - Epinephrine raises glucose levels
  - Blockade → hypoglycemia
- Blockade of hypoglycemia symptoms
  - ↓ glucose → sweating/tachycardia
  - Symptoms "masked" by beta blockers

Beta Blockers
Side effects

- Caution in **asthma/COPD**
  - β2 receptors: bronchodilators
  - β2 blockade may cause a flare
  - β1 blockers ("cardioselective") often used
- Decompensated **heart failure**
  - β1 blockers lower cardiac output → worsening of symptoms
  - Commonly used in compensated heart failure
  - Mortality benefit

Beta Blockers
Overdose

- Depression of myocardial contractility → shock
- Bradycardia/AV block

Beta Blockers
Overdose

- Treatment: Glucagon
  - Activates adenyl cyclase at different site from beta receptors
  - ↑ cAMP → ↑ intracellular Ca
  - Increased contraction and heart rate

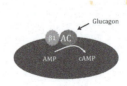

α1 Blockers
Tamsulosin, Alfuzosin, Doxazosin, Terazosin

- α1 receptors in periphery: vasoconstrict
- Blockade → vasodilation → ↓TPR → ↓BP
- Used in benign prostatic hypertrophy
  - Relax smooth muscle of bladder/prostate
  - Increase urine flow
- Common side effect: Postural hypotension
- Tamsulosin: "Uroselective"
  - Less hypotension effect

Alpha 2 Receptors

α2 receptors in CNS
Presynaptic receptor   Feedback to nerve when NE released
Activation leads to ↓NE release

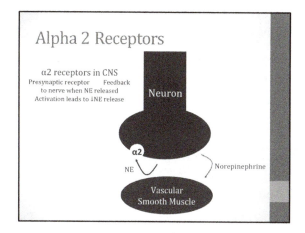

Clonidine
α2 agonist

- Old, rarely used hypertension drug
- Key side effect: Rebound hypertension
  - Abrupt cessation of drug (usually at high dose)
  - Severe hypertension (SBP>200; DBP>120)
  - Symptoms of high BP and sympathetic over-activity
  - Nervousness, sweating, headache, chest pain
- Also causes sedation

Methyldopa
α2 agonist

- Drug of choice in pregnancy
- Also causes sedation
- Key side effect (rare): Hemolytic anemia

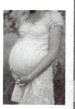
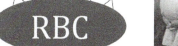

Calcium Channel Blockers

- Three major classes of calcium antagonists
  - dihydropyridines (nifedipine)
  - phenylalkylamines (verapamil)
  - benzothiazepines (diltiazem)
- **Vasodilators** and negative chronotropes/inotropes

Calcium Channel Blockers

- Vascular smooth muscle effects
  - Nifedipine>Diltiazem>Verapamil
- Heart rate/contractility effects
  - Verapamil>Diltiazem>Nifedipine

Calcium Channel Blockers

- **Dihydropyridines (nifedipine)** → vasodilators
  - Main effect: ↓TPR
- **Non-dihydropyridines (Verapamil, diltiazem)**
  - Similar to β1 blockers
  - Main effects: ↓HR; ↓contractility

Calcium Channel Blockers
Dihydropyridines (nifedipine)

- Used for hypertension
- Flushing, headache, hypotension
  - Peripheral vasodilation
- Key side effect: edema
  - Increased *capillary* hydrostatic pressure
  - Pre-capillary arteriolar vasodilation

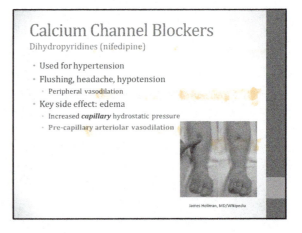

Calcium Channel Blockers
Dihydropyridines (nifedipine)

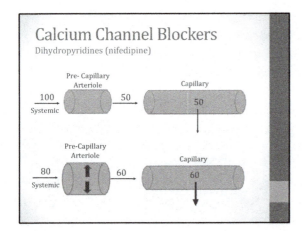

Calcium Channel Blockers
Verapamil, diltiazem

- Used for hypertension
- Also used in heart disease
  - Arrhythmias (atrial fibrillation)
  - Stable angina (lower oxygen demand)
- Potential side effect: Negative inotropes
  - Can precipitate heart failure

Calcium Channel Blockers
Other Side Effects

- Constipation
  - Most commonly with verapamil

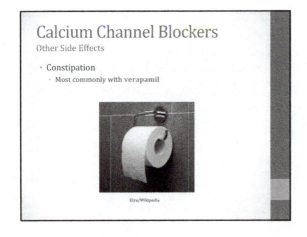

Calcium Channel Blockers
Other Side Effects

- Hyperprolactinemia
  - Seen with verapamil
  - Blocks calcium channels CNS → ↓ dopamine release
  - Causes hypogonadism
  - Men: ↓ libido, impotence
  - Pre-menopausal women: irregular menses, galactorrhea

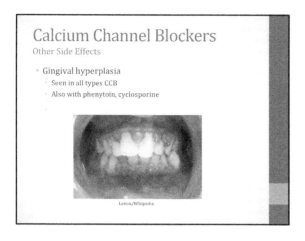
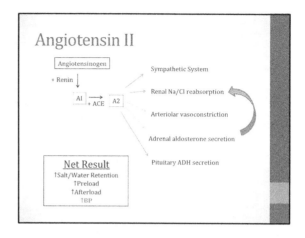
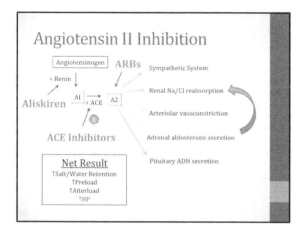
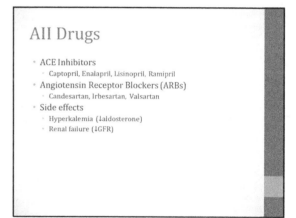
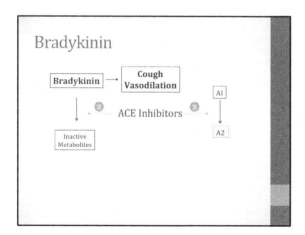
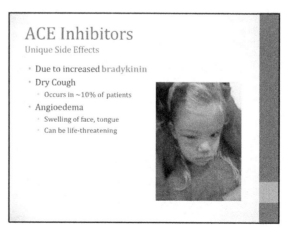

Aliskiren

- Direct renin inhibitor
- Reduces angiotensin I levels (unique effect)

Angiotensinogen
+ Renin ↓
AI →(+ ACE) A2

Diuretics

- Loop diuretics
  - Furosemide, bumetanide, torsemide, ethacrynic acid
- Thiazide diuretics
  - Hydrochlorothiazide; chlorthalidone; metolazone
- Potassium sparing diuretics
  - Spironolactone, Eplerenone, Triamterene, Amiloride

Hydralazine

- Direct arteriolar vasodilator
- Rarely used for hypertension
- Combined with nitrates for heart failure
- Safe in pregnancy
- Causes drug-induced lupus

Drug-induced Lupus

- Syndrome similar to lupus
  - Often rash, arthritis, low blood cell counts
  - Milder than SLE
  - Usually no associated renal failure/CNS disease
- Key finding: anti-histone antibodies
- Three drugs
  - Hydralazine
  - Procainamide
  - Isoniazid

Hypertensive Emergency

- Unique drugs used for therapy
  - Intravenous, rapid acting
- Lowering BP too fast can cause ischemia
  - Autoregulation of vascular beds → vasoconstriction

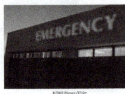

Hypertensive Emergency

- Nitroprusside
  - Short acting drug
  - ↑ intracellular cGMP
  - ↑ nitric oxide release
  - Venous and arteriolar vasodilation
  - ↓ preload (VR); ↓ afterload
- Cyanide toxicity with prolonged use
  - Multiple cyanide groups per molecule
  - Inhibits electron transport
  - Toxic levels with prolonged infusions

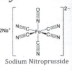
Sodium Nitroprusside

Hypertensive Emergency

- Fenoldopam
  - D1 agonist
  - Arteriolar vasodilation
  - Increased urinary sodium/water excretion
  - Maintains renal perfusion while vasodilating

Hypertensive Emergency

- Labetalol
  - β1 and α1 Blocker
- Esmolol
  - Rapid acting intravenous β1 blocker
- Nicardipine, Clevidipine
  - Intravenous dihydropyridine calcium channel blocker

Orthostatic Hypotension
Postural Hypotension; Orthostasis

- ↓blood pressure due to gravity with standing
- Compensation from **sympathetic nervous system**
  - Increased VR, CO, HR, TPR
  - Impaired with low volume, low TPR, blunted ANS
- Severe ↓BP (>20mmHg) = orthostatic hypotension
  - Dizziness, syncope
- Common etiologies:
  - Hypovolemia
  - Hypertensive medications

Orthostatic Hypotension
Postural Hypotension; Orthostasis

- Alpha-1 blockers
- ACE-inhibitors
  - Especially in patients on diuretics
  - Volume depletion → ↑RAAS
  - "First dose hypotension"

Reflex Tachycardia

- Vasodilation → ↓BP → ↑SNS
- Reflex response: ↑ HR
- Can be caused by vasodilators
  - Hydralazine
  - Alpha-1 blockers
  - Dihydropyridine calcium channel blockers
  - Nitroglycerine
- May exacerbate chronic stable angina
- Drugs may be co-administered with β blocker

Choosing Drugs

- Diabetes
  - ACE inhibitors: Protective of kidneys
  - Beta blockers can lower glucose and mask hypoglycemia
  - HCTZ can increase glucose
- Systolic Heart Failure
  - ACEi, beta blockers, aldosterone blockers: mortality benefit
  - Calcium channel blockers → ↓ contractility

Choosing Drugs

- Hypertension in Pregnancy
  - Methyldopa
  - Beta blockers, nifedipine, hydralazine
  - Avoid: ACE inhibitors, ARBs, direct renin inhibitors
  - Associated with congenital malformations
- Significant renal failure or ↑K
  - Avoid: ACE-inhibitors, ARBs (↓AII, ↓aldsoterone)
  - Avoid: Potassium sparing diuretics (↑ K)
  - Avoid: Other diuretics (↓ECV → ↓GFR)
  - Calcium blockers, beta blockers usually ok

Valve Disease

Jason Ryan, MD, MPH

Heart Valves

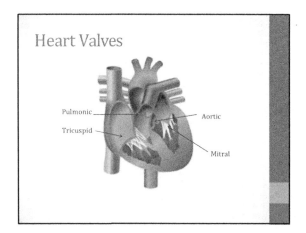

Pulmonic, Tricuspid, Aortic, Mitral

Valve Disease

- Stenosis
  - Stiffening/thickening of valve leaflets
  - Obstruction to forward blood flow
- **Regurgitation**
  - Malcoaptation of valve leaflets
  - Leakage of blood flow backwards across valve

Valve Lesions - Systole

- Occur when heart contracts/squeezes
- Aortic stenosis
- Mitral regurgitation
- Pulmonic stenosis
- Tricuspid regurgitation

Valve Lesions - Diastole

- Occur when heart relaxes/fills
- Aortic regurgitation
- Mitral stenosis
- Pulmonic regurgitation
- Tricuspid stenosis

Valve Disorders
Treatments

- Only severe valvular lesions treated
- Mostly surgical diseases
- Surgical repair
  - Often done for mitral valve prolapse → mitral regurgitation
- Valve replacement
  - Bioprosthetic (pig or cow)
  - Mechanical (requires life-long anticoagulation)
- Valvuloplasty (stenotic lesions)

Stenotic Valve Disorders

- Stiff valve
- "Gradient" across valve
- High pressure upstream
- Lower pressure downstream

Rheumatic Fever

- Occurs weeks after **streptococcal pharyngitis**
- Common in **children**
- Autoimmune: type II hypersensitivity reaction
- Antibodies to bacterial **M proteins** cross-react

Rheumatic Fever

- Jones criteria
  - Joints: Polyarthritis (>5 joints)
  - ♥: Carditis (valvulitis, myocarditis, pericarditis)
  - Nodules (subcutaneous)
  - Erythema marginatum (rash on trunk)
  - Sydenham chorea (jerking movement disorder)

Rheumatic Heart Disease

- Damage to heart valves by rheumatic fever
- **Mitral valve** most commonly involved
- Often presents years after acute rheumatic fever
- Many patients do not recall acute symptoms
- Common in **developing countries**
  - Limited access to medical care for pharyngitis
  - Often seen in **immigrants to US**

Carcinoid Heart Disease

- Caused by carcinoid tumors of intestines
- Secrete serotonin
- Fibrous deposits **tricuspid/pulmonic valves**
- Leads to stenosis and regurgitation
- Serotonin inactivated by lungs
- Left sided lesions rare

Aortic Stenosis
Pathophysiology

- Stiff aortic valve
- Systolic problem
- **Increased afterload**

Aortic Stenosis
Hemodynamics

- LV pressure systolic >> aortic pressure
  - LVSP = 160mmHg (normal = 120)
  - SBP = 120mmHg (normal = 120)
  - Gradient = 40mmHg
- ↑ **LVEDP** due to ↑ afterload

Aortic Stenosis
Clinical features

- Systolic crescendo-decrescendo murmur
- **Syncope**: failure to ↑CO due to ↑ afterload
- **Angina**: ↑ LVEDP → ↓ coronary blood flow
- **Left heart failure**: ↑ LVEDP

Aortic Stenosis
Causes

- **Senile aortic stenosis**
  - "Wear and tear"
  - Collagen breakdown
  - Calcium deposition
- Bicuspid aortic valve
- Rarely rheumatic heart disease

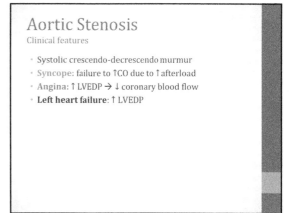

Supravalvular Aortic Stenosis

- Narrowing of ascending aorta above aortic valve
- Seen in Williams syndrome
- Genetic deletion syndrome

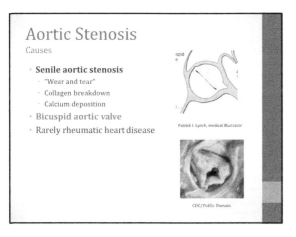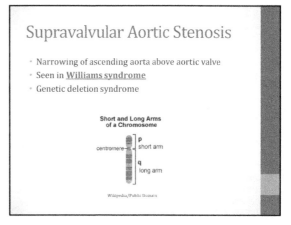

Mitral Stenosis
Pathophysiology

- Stiff mitral valve
- Diastolic problem
- LA pressure >> LV diastolic pressure
  - Left atrial pressure 20mmHg (normal = 10)
  - LVEDP 5mmHg (normal = 10)
  - Gradient = 15mmHg
- **Decreased preload**

Mitral Stenosis
Clinical features

- Caused by **rheumatic fever**
- Most common symptom: dyspnea
  - ↑ LA pressure → pulmonary congestion
- Murmur: diastolic rumble with opening snap

Tricuspid Stenosis

- Very rare valve disorder
- Diastolic murmur at left lower sternal border
- Caused by rheumatic fever (with mitral disease)
  - Tricuspid regurgitation more common
- Carcinoid heart disease

Pulmonic Stenosis

- Congenital defect in children
  - Fused commissures with thickened leaflets
- Carcinoid heart disease

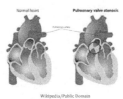

Wikipedia/Public Domain

Regurgitant Lesions

- Acute and chronic forms
- Acute regurgitation (often from endocarditis)
  - May cause shock
  - Activation of sympathetic nervous system
  - Increased contractility
  - Increased afterload
- Chronic regurgitation
  - No shock
  - Leads to chronic heart failure
  - Sympathetic activation only if severe heart failure

Aortic Regurgitation
Pathophysiology

- Blood leaks across aortic valve
- Diastolic problem
- **Increased preload, stroke volume**
- Increased afterload
  - More stroke volume → aorta → ↓ compliance (stiffening)
- Blowing diastolic murmur

Aortic Regurgitation
Causes

- **Dilated aortic root → leaflets pull apart**
  - Often from HTN or other aortic aneurysm
  - Rarely from tertiary syphilis (aortitis)
- Bicuspid aortic valve
  - Turner syndrome
  - Coarctation of the aorta
- Endocarditis
- Rheumatic heart disease
  - Almost always with mitral disease

Aortic Regurgitation
Clinical features

- Leaking blood back into LV causes low diastolic BP
  - 120/80 (normal) → 120/40
  - Low diastolic pressure
- Wide pulse pressure
  - High cardiac output with low diastolic pressure
- Wide pulse pressure symptoms
  - "Water hammer" pulses
  - Head bobbing
  - Many, many others (mostly historical)

Mitral Regurgitation
Pathophysiology

- Blood leaks across mitral valve
- Increased LA volume → Starling mechanism
- Increased left ventricular filling from LA
- **Increased preload, stroke volume**
- Reduced afterload

Mitral Regurgitation
Causes

- Primary MR caused by **mitral valve prolapse**
  - Also called degenerative or myxomatous
- Billowing of mitral valve leaflets above annulus
- Common cause of **mitral regurgitation**
- Causes a **systolic click**
  - Don't confuse with opening snap of mitral stenosis

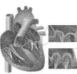

Mitral Regurgitation
Secondary causes

- Ischemia → damage to papillary muscle
- Left ventricular dilation
  - Dilated cardiomyopathy
  - Leaflets pulled apart
  - "Functional" MR
- Hypertrophic cardiomyopathy

Mitral Regurgitation
Causes

- Endocarditis
- Rheumatic heart disease
- Congenital
  - Cleft mitral valve
  - Endocardial cushion defect
  - Down syndrome

Mitral Regurgitation
Clinical Features

- Holosystolic murmur at apex

Afterload Reduction
Aortic and Mitral Regurgitation

- In theory, ↓ afterload can improve forward flow
- For severe, acute regurgitation this helps
- For chronic disease, clinical trials with mixed results
- In general, these are surgical diseases
- Common test scenario "Best medical option?"

Tricuspid Regurgitation

- Small amount of TR normal ("physiologic TR")
- Holosystolic murmur at left sternal border
- Pathologic causes
  - Functional TR from RV enlargement
  - Endocarditis - classically IV drug users
  - Carcinoid
  - Ebstein's anomaly

Pulmonic Regurgitation

- Most common cause: repaired **Tetralogy of Fallot**
  - Repair of RVOT obstruction damages valve
- Endocarditis (rare)
- Rheumatic heart disease (rare)

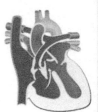

Tetralogy of Fallot

Shock

Jason Ryan, MD, MPH

Shock

- Life-threatening fall in blood pressure
- Poor tissue perfusion
- Low cardiac output
  - Loss of contractility
  - Low intravascular volume
- Peripheral vasodilation

$$BP = CO \times TPR$$

Types of Shock

- Cardiogenic
  - Cardiac disorder → fall in cardiac output
- Hypovolemic
  - Fall in intravascular volume → fall in cardiac output
  - Hemorrhage
- Distributive
  - Peripheral vasodilation
  - Septic, anaphylactic
- Obstructive

Types of Shock

- Different treatments for different types of shock
- Often can determine type from history
  - Myocardial infarction → cardiogenic shock
  - Massive bleeding → hypovolemic shock
- Shock of unclear etiology: Swan-Ganz catheter

Swan-Ganz Catheter
Pulmonary artery catheter

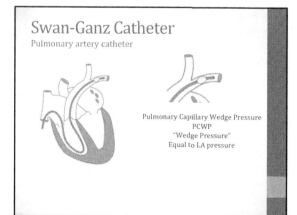

Pulmonary Capillary Wedge Pressure
PCWP
"Wedge Pressure"
Equal to LA pressure

Swan-Ganz Data

- RA Pressure (Normal ~ 5mmHg)
- RV Pressure (20/5)
- PA Pressure (20/10)
- PCWP Pressure (10)
- Mixed venous O2 sat
  - Oxygen concentration after all veins mix

Fick Equation

Oxygen Consumed = O2 Out Lungs – O2 In Lungs
= CO (Art O2 – Ven O2)

$$\text{Cardiac Output} = \frac{\text{O2 Consumption}}{(\text{Art O2} - \text{Ven O2})}$$

O2 Consumption α body size   Arterial
O2 Content = O2 sat on finger probe   Venous
O2 Content = O2 from Swan-Ganz

Swan-Ganz catheter gives cardiac output

Flow Equation

- Used to determine systemic vascular resistance

$$\Delta P = CO * SVR \quad \text{MAP}$$
$$- RAP = CO * SVR$$

$$SVR = \frac{MAP - RAP}{CO}$$

Swan-Ganz Catheter gives SVR

Swan-Ganz Data

- Direct
  - RA Pressure (Normal ~ 5mmHg)
  - RV Pressure (20/5)
  - PA Pressure (20/10)
  - PCWP Pressure (10)
  - Mixed venous O2 sat
- Calculated
  - Cardiac output
  - Systemic Vascular Resistance

Hemodynamic of Shock

- Four major classes of shock
- All have different hemodynamics from Swan
- Swan can be used to determine etiology of shock
  - Cardiogenic
  - Hypovolemic
  - Distributive
  - Obstructive

Cardiogenic Shock

- Hallmark is low cardiac output
- **High cardiac pressures**
- High SVR (sympathetic response)
- Classic cause: large myocardial infarction
- Also seen in advanced heart failure (depressed LVEF)

Hypovolemic Shock

- Poor fluid intake
- High fever, insensible losses
- Hemorrhage
- Low cardiac output
- **Low cardiac pressures**
- High SVR (sympathetic response)

Distributive Shock

- Hallmark is low SVR
- Diffuse vasodilation and/or endothelial dysfunction
- Sepsis (most common)
- Anaphylaxis
- Neurogenic
- Cardiac output classically high (variable)
- Cardiac pressures variable

Type of Shock

	Cardiogenic	Hypovolemic	Distributive
Blood Pressure	↓	↓	↓
HR	↑	↑	↑
RA Pressure	↑	↓	↓/-
RV Pressure	↑	↓	↓/-
PCWP	↑	↓	↓/-
Cardiac Output	↓	↓	↑
SVR	↑	↑	↓

Major Shock Types

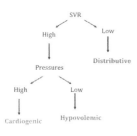

Physical Exam

- Cold skin → high SVR and low CO
  - Cardiogenic
  - Hypovolemic
- Warm skin → low SVR and high CO
  - Distributive
- Jugular venous pressure → high RA pressure
- Pulmonary rales → high LA pressure

Obstructive Shock

- Obstruction to blood flow from heart
- Low cardiac output despite normal contractility
- Tamponade
- Tension pneumothorax
- Massive pulmonary embolism
- Low cardiac output
- High SVR

Treatment of Shock

- Cardiogenic: inotropes
  - Milrinone, Dobutamine
- Hypovolemic: volume
  - Blood transfusions, IV fluids
- Distributive: vasopressors
  - Phenylephrine, epinephrine, norepinephrine
- Obstructive: resolve obstruction
  - Treat tamponade, embolism, tension pneumothorax

Swan in Valve Disease

RA (5)	15
RV (20/5)	45/15
PA (20/10)	45/30
PCWP (10)	30
LV (120/10)	120/5
Ao (120/80)	120/80

Mitral Stenosis

Swan in Valve Disease

RA (5)	5
RV (20/5)	20/5
PA (20/10)	20/10
PCWP (10)	10
LV (120/10)	150/10
Ao (120/80)	120/80

Aortic Stenosis

Swan in Valve Disease

RA (5)	15
RV (20/5)	45/15
PA (20/10)	45/30
PCWP (10)	30
LV (120/10)	120/30
Ao (120/80)	120/40

Aortic Regurgitation

Left Atrial Pressure

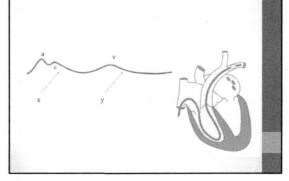

Giant V waves

- Seen in **mitral regurgitation** in PCPW tracing
- Similar to giant V waves in tricuspid regurgitation
  - Seen in venous pressure tracing

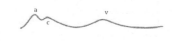

Pericardial Disease

Jason Ryan MD, MPH

Pericardium

- Three layers
- Fibrous pericardium
- Serous pericardium
  - Parietal layer
  - Visceral layer
- Pericardial cavity between serous layers
- Innervated by phrenic nerve
- Pericarditis → referred pain to the shoulder

Pericardial Diseases

- Pericarditis
- Tamponade
- Constrictive pericarditis

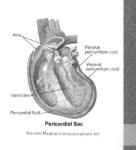

Pericarditis

- Most common pericardial disorder
- Inflammation of the pericardium
- Immune-mediated (details not known)
- May recur after treatment

Pericarditis
Clinical Features

- Chest pain
  - Sharp
  - Worse with deep breath (pleuritic)
  - Worse lying flat (supine)
  - Better sitting up/leaning forward
- Fever
- Leukocytosis
- Elevated ESR

Pericarditis
EKG Findings

Pericarditis
EKG Findings

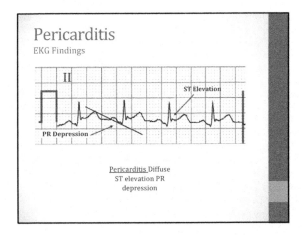

Pericarditis Diffuse ST elevation PR depression

Pericarditis
EKG

- Technically, 4 stages of EKG changes
- Stage 1: diffuse ST elevations, PR depressions
- Stage 2 (~1 week later): Normal
- Stage 3: T wave inversions
- Stage 4: Normal

Pericarditis
Physical Exam

- Pericardial friction rub
- Scratchy sound
- Systole and diastole

Pericarditis
Etiology

- Usually idiopathic
- Viral
  - Classic cause is Coxsackievirus
  - Often follows viral upper respiratory infection (URI)
- Bacterial
  - Spread of pneumonia
  - Complication of surgery
  - Tuberculosis
- Fungal

Pericarditis
Etiology

- Uremic (renal failure)
- Post-myocardial infarction
  - Fibrinous (days after MI)
  - Dressler's syndrome (weeks after MI)
- Autoimmune disease (RA, Lupus)

Pericarditis
Treatment

- NSAIDs
- Steroids
- Colchicine
  - Inhibits WBCs via complex mechanism
  - Useful in gout and familial Mediterranean fever
  - Added to NSAIDs to lower risk of recurrence

Myopericarditis

- Myocarditis = inflammation of myocardium
- Similar presentation to ischemia
  - Chest pain
  - EKG changes
  - Increased CK-MB, Troponin

Tamponade

- Accumulation of pericardial fluid
- High pericardial pressure
- Filling restriction of cardiac chambers
- Amount of fluid variable
  - Acute accumulation (bleeding): small amount of fluid
  - Chronic accumulation (cancer): large amount of fluid

Tamponade

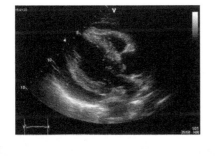

Water Bottle Sign

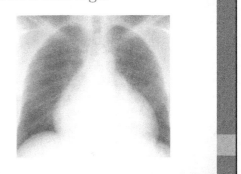

Tamponade
Causes

- Cancer metastases to pericardium
- Uremia
- Pericarditis
- Trauma
- Treatment: Drainage of effusion

Tamponade
Clinical features

- Distant heart sounds
- Dyspnea
  - High left atrial pressure
  - Pulmonary edema
- Elevated jugular venous pressure

Tamponade
Clinical features

- Beck's Triad
  - Distant heart sounds
  - Elevated JVP
  - Hypotension
- Seen in rapidly-developing traumatic effusions
- Severe impairment LV function → low cardiac output
- Slower effusions: Pericardium stretches/dilates

Pulsus Paradoxus

- Classic finding in tamponade
- Systolic BP always falls slightly on inspiration
- Exaggerated fall (>10mmHg) = pulsus paradoxus
- Severe fall = pulse disappears

Pulsus Paradoxus

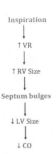

Inspiration
↓
↑ VR
↓
↑ RV Size
↓
Septum bulges
↓
↓ LV Size
↓
↓ CO

Pulsus Paradoxus

- Also seen in **asthma and COPD**
- Inspiration: ↓ left sided flow
- Caused by pulmonary pressure fluctuation
- Exaggerated in lung disease
  - Normal lungs: 0 to -5mmHg
  - Lung disease: Change up to 40mmHg
- Large drop in left sided flow → pulsus paradoxus

Pulsus Paradoxus
Measurement Technique

- Raise cuff pressure until no sounds heard
- **NORMAL respirations**
- Slowly lower cuff pressure
- First point (P1): intermittent sounds
- Second point (P2): constant sounds
- Pulsus = P1 – P2

Tamponade
EKG

- Sinus tachycardia
- Low voltage – EKG sees less electricity due to effusion

Electrical Alternans

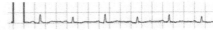

Tamponade
Prominent x descent, Blunted y descent

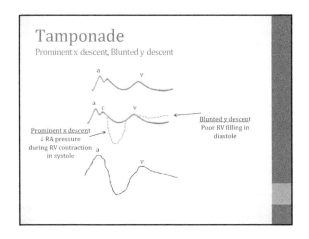

Equalization of Pressures

- Occurs when cardiac chambers cannot relax
- Pressure in RA, RV, LA, LV falls but then abruptly stops
- Seen in tamponade and pericardial constriction

Parameter	Normal	Tamponade
RA mean	5	20
RV Pressure	20/5	44/20
PCPW Pressure	10	20

Constrictive Pericarditis

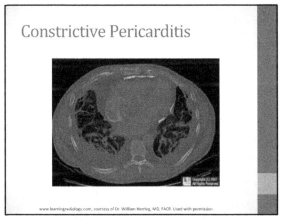

www.learningradiology.com, courtesy of Dr. William Herring, MD, FACR. Used with permission.

Constrictive Pericarditis

- Fibrous, calcified scar in pericardium
- Loss of elasticity: stiff, thickened, sticky
- Can result from many pericardial disease processes
  - Pericarditis
  - Radiation to chest
  - Heart surgery

Constrictive Pericarditis
Clinical Features

- Dyspnea
- Prominent **right heart failure**
  - Markedly elevated jugular venous pressure
  - Lower extremity edema
  - Liver congestion
  - May lead to cirrhosis ("nutmeg liver")

David Monniaux/Wikipedia

Constrictive Pericarditis
Other Features

- Pulsus paradoxus uncommon (~20%)
- High RA, RVEDP, PCPW pressures
- Equalization of pressures
- Pericardial knock

S1   S2
         Pericardial
         Knock

Kussmaul's Sign

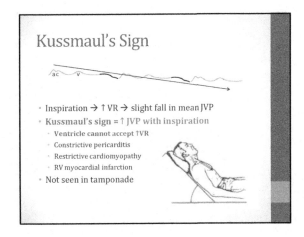

- Inspiration → ↑VR → slight fall in mean JVP
- **Kussmaul's sign = ↑ JVP with inspiration**
  - Ventricle cannot accept ↑VR
  - Constrictive pericarditis
  - Restrictive cardiomyopathy
  - RV myocardial infarction
- Not seen in tamponade

Pulsus and Kussmaul's

- Pulsus paradoxus: classic sign of tamponade
  - Pulsus in tamPonade
- Kussmaul's sign: classic sign of constriction
  - Also seen in restrictive heart disease
  - Kussmaul's in Konstriction/Restriction

	Tamponade	Constriction	Restrictive
Pulsus	Yes	No	No
Kussmaul's	No	Yes	Yes

Constrictive Pericarditis
Rapid/prominent y descent

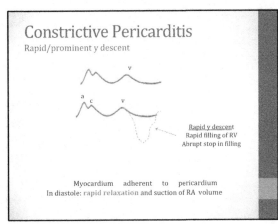

Rapid y descent
Rapid filling of RV
Abrupt stop in filling

Myocardium adherent to pericardium
In diastole: rapid relaxation and suction of RA volume

Venous Pressure Findings

	Tamponade	Constriction
x descent	Rapid	--
y descent	Absent	Rapid

Dip and Plateau
Square Root Sign

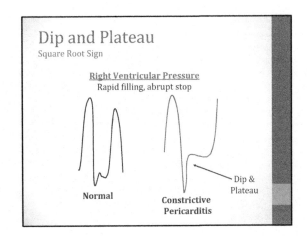

Right Ventricular Pressure
Rapid filling, abrupt stop

Normal | Constrictive Pericarditis | Dip & Plateau

Constriction and Restriction

- Constrictive pericarditis/Restrictive heart disease
- Many common features
- Prominent right heart failure
- Kussmaul's sign
- Rapid y descent
- Dip and plateau

Aortic Dissection

Jason Ryan, MD, MPH

Aortic Dissection
CT Angiogram

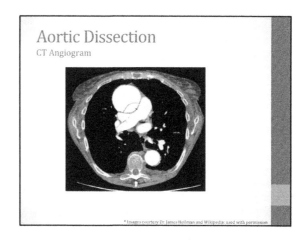

*Images courtesy Dr. James Heilman and Wikipedia; used with permission

Aortic Dissection

- Three layers to aorta
  - Intima
  - Media
  - Adventicia
- Dissection → tear in intima
- Blood "dissects" intima and media

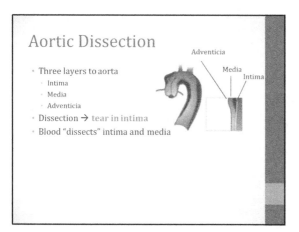

Propagation

- Blood enters dissection plane
- Spreads proximal, distal
- Can disrupt flow to vessels

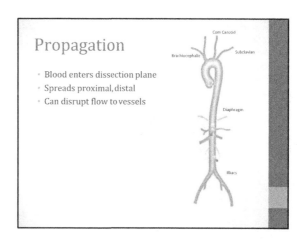

Types

- Type A
  - Involves ascending aorta and/or arch
  - Treated surgically
- Type B
  - Descending aorta
  - Can be treated medically
  - Control hypertension/symptoms
  - Surgical mortality high

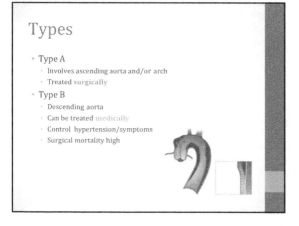

Symptoms

- "Tearing" chest pain radiating to back

Other symptoms

- Propagation to aortic root
  - Aortic regurgitation
  - Pericardial effusion/tamponade
  - Myocardial ischemia (obstruction RCA origin)
- Propagation to aortic arch
  - Stroke (carotids)
  - Horner's syndrome
  - Vocal cord paralysis

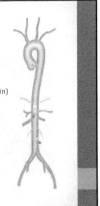

Recurrent Laryngeal Nerve

- Branch of vagus nerve
- Supplies larynx and voice box
- Compression:
  - Aortic dissection
  - Massive left atrial enlargement

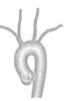

Other findings

- **Blood pressure differential** between arms
- **Widened mediastinum** on chest x-ray

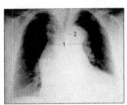

JHeuser /Wikipedia

Diagnosis

- Suggested by history, exam, chest x-ray
- Definitive diagnosis
  - CT scan
  - MRI
  - Transesophageal echocardiogram (TEE)
- D-dimer
  - Sensitive but not specific
  - Normal value makes aortic dissection unlikely

Risk Factors
General Principles

- Medial layer of aorta
  - Tensile strength and elasticity
  - Key proteins: collagen and elastin
  - Weakness of medial layer → dissection/aneurysms
  - Common aneurysm feature: medial damage/destruction
- Vasa vasorum
  - Network of small vessels primarily in adventitial layer
  - Supplies blood to medial layer in thick vessels (i.e. aorta)
  - Thickening (HTN) → weakening of medial layer

Risk Factors
General Principles

- Requires **tension** on wall
  - Common in proximal aorta (near aortic valve)
  - High tension from blood moving out of heart
  - Worsened by hypertension
- Requires weakness of media layer
  - Also caused by hypertension
  - Seen in collagen disorders (genetic)

Risk Factors
General Principles

- **Cystic medial necrosis**
  - Development of cysts and necrosis in medial layer
- Occurs to mild degree with aging
- More rapid with:
  - Bicuspid aortic valve
  - Marfan syndrome
- Common in **ascending thoracic aneurysms**

Risk Factors
Aortic Dissection

- Aortic damage
  - HTN - #1 risk factor
  - Atherosclerosis
  - Thoracic aneurysm
- Abnormal collagen
  - Marfan Syndrome
  - Ehlers-Danlos
- Others
  - Bicuspid aortic valve
  - Turner Syndrome (bicuspid, coarctation)
  - Tertiary syphilis: Aortitis

Aortic Aneurysms

- Dilation/bulge of aorta
- More than 1.5x normal
- Involves all three 3 layers
- Thoracic (TAAs)
- Abdominal (AAAs)

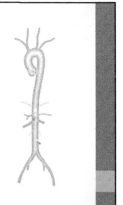

Thoracic Aortic Aneurysms

- Important risk factor for dissection
- Usually occur in proximal/ascending aorta
- Usually seen in association with another disorder
  - Marfan, Turner, Bicuspid aortic valve, Syphilis
- Family history of aneurysm important
- May be associated with atherosclerosis
  - More common in descending aorta
  - Occur in association with atherosclerosis risk factors
  - HTN, smoking, high cholesterol

Thoracic Aortic Aneurysms
Symptoms

- Most are asymptomatic
- Can cause **aortic regurgitation**
- Surgery if size >5.0cm

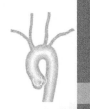

Abdominal Aortic Aneurysms

- More common than thoracic aneurysms
- Classically taught as a disease of atherosclerosis
- Infrarenal aorta most affected by atherosclerosis
- Also most common site of AAA
- Current research suggests many factors
  - Genetic, environmental, hemodynamic, immunologic

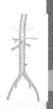

Abdominal Aortic Aneurysms
Risk Factors

- **Smoking**: strongest association with AAA
- **Males**: 10x more common men vs. women
- Age
  - Rare before 55
  - As high as 5% in men >65
- HTN, hyperlipidemia

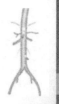

Abdominal Aortic Aneurysms

- Most are asymptomatic
- Some detected on physical exam
- **Pulsatile mass** from xiphoid to umbilicus
- Natural history is enlargement → rupture
- Followed with **ultrasound** or CT scan
- Surgery if >5.0cm

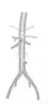

Aortic Rupture

- Usually from trauma
- Most common site is isthmus

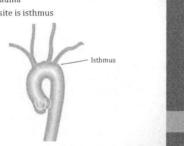

Cardiac Tumors

Jason Ryan, MD, MPH

Cardiac Tumors

- Myxoma
  - Most common 1° cardiac tumor
- Rhabdomyomas
  - Most common 1° cardiac tumor children
- Metastatic tumors
  - Most common cardiac tumor overall

Myxoma

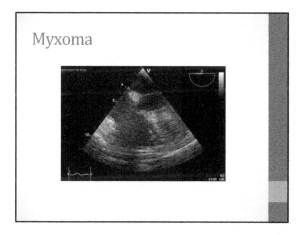

Myxoma

- Common in the left atrium (80%)
  - Usually attached to atrial septum
  - Often at the border of fossa ovalis
- Benign (do not metastasize)

Myxoma

- Mesenchymal cells (undifferentiated cells)
- Endothelial cells
- Thrombus/clot
- Mucopolysaccharides

Myxoma

- Often cause systemic symptoms
  - "B symptoms"
  - Fevers, chills, sweats
- Can embolize → stroke

Myxoma

- May disrupt mitral valve function
  - Regurgitation
  - Heart failure
- Can sit in mitral valve
  - "Ball in valve"
  - Mitral stenosis symptoms
  - Syncope or sudden death
- Auscultation: Diastolic "tumor plop"

Cardiac Rhabdomyomas

- Tumors of muscle cells
- Benign (do not metastasize)
- Usually children (most <1year)
- Sometimes detected prenatal
- Tumor embedded in ventricular wall
- Most regress spontaneously
- Rare symptoms from obstruction of blood flow

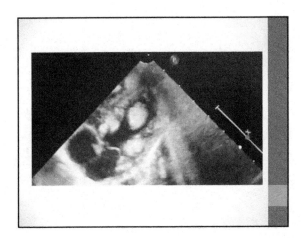

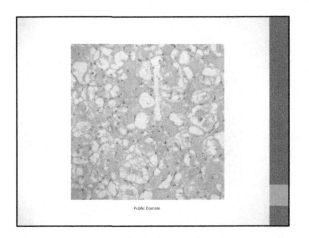

Public Domain

Cardiac Rhabdomyomas

- Associated with tuberous sclerosis (90%)
- Autosomal dominant genetic syndrome
- Mutation in TSC1 or TSC2 gene
- TSC1: Hamartin
- TSC2: Tuberin
- Mutations → widespread tumor formation

Tuberous Sclerosis

- Involves MULTIPLE organ systems
- Numerous hamartomas and other neoplasms
- Seizures – most common presenting feature
- "Ash leaf spots": Pale, hypopigmented skin lesions
- Facial skin spots (angiofibromas)
- Mental retardation

Tuberous Sclerosis

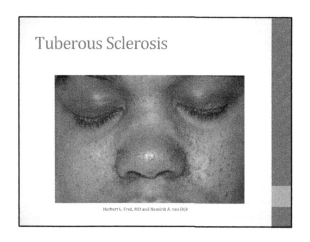

Tuberous Sclerosis

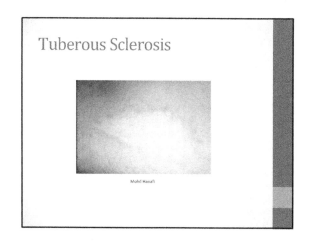

Hypertrophic Cardiomyopathy

Jason Ryan, MD, MPH

Hypertrophic Cardiomyopathy

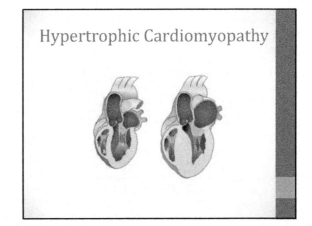

Hypertrophic Cardiomyopathy
Names

- Hypertrophic cardiomyopathy (HCM)
- Hypertrophic obstructive cardiomyopathy (HOCM)
- Idiopathic hypertrophic subaortic stenosis (IHSS)

HCM

- Genetic disorder caused by gene mutations
- About 50% cases familial (50% sporadic)
- Autosomal dominant
- Variable expression
  - Significant variation in severity of symptoms
  - Many variations in location/severity of hypertrophy

Wikipedia/Public Domain

Morphologic Variants

- Subaortic
- Midventricular
- Apical
- Diffuse

Zorkun/Wikipedia

HCM

- Often **single-point missense mutations**
  - Point mutation → altered amino acid in protein
  - 15+ genes with 1500+ mutations identified
- Often involve genes for **cardiac sarcomere proteins**
  - Beta-myosin heavy chain (40% cases)
  - Myosin binding protein (40% cases)

HCM
Histology

- Myocyte disarray (excessive branching)
- Hypertrophy
- Interstitial fibrosis

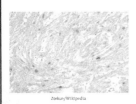
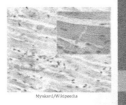

HCM
Clinical Features

- Many patients asymptomatic
- Heart failure
  - Diastolic dysfunction
  - Impaired emptying due to LVOT obstruction
- **Chest pain (angina)**
  - Increased O2 demand

HCM
Clinical Features

- Sudden cardiac death
  - Abnormal myocytes → ventricular arrhythmias
  - Most common cause SCD in young patients
- **Syncope**
  - Arrhythmias may lead to syncope
  - Thickened myocardium → LVOT obstruction
- **Mitral regurgitation**

HCM
Clinical Features

- Problem #1: Arrhythmia problem
  - Thick myocardium vulnerable to arrhythmias
  - Most serious is ventricular tachycardia → sudden death
  - Exercise (catecholamines) increase risk SCD
  - Sudden death in athletes
  - Defibrillators for high risk patients
  - Avoidance of exercise

HCM
Clinical Features

- Problem #2: Outflow obstruction problem
  - Thickened myocardium obstructs blood leaving LV
  - Same physics and symptoms as aortic stenosis
  - Heart failure, chest pain, exercise-induced syncope
  - Treated with surgery
  - Beta blockers (↓ contractility)
  - Ca blockers (verapamil)

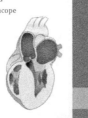

HCM
Clinical Features

- #3: Mitral valve problem
  - High velocity in LVOT tugs mitral valve chords and leaflets
  - Causes systolic anterior motion (SAM) of mitral valve
  - Over time this leads to mitral regurgitation

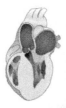

HCM
Clinical Features

- Systolic ejection murmur
- Caused by outflow tract obstruction
- Sounds just like AS unless you do maneuvers
- Lots of associated abnormal heart sounds
  - S4
  - Holosystolic murmur of MR
  - Paradoxical split S2

S1   S2

HCM
Maneuvers

- For any HCM maneuver, think about size of LV
- ↑ LV size → ↓ murmur
- ↓ LV size → ↑ murmur

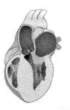

HCM
Maneuvers

- Valsalva
  - Patient bears down as if having a bowel movement
  - Or blows out against closed glottis
  - Increase thoracic pressure → compression of veins → ↓VR
  - Less VR → Less preload → Smaller LV cavity
  - Obstructing septum moves further into the outflow tract
  - Murmur **INCREASES** in intensity

HCM
Maneuvers

- Squatting
  - Forces blood volume stored in legs to return to heart
  - Preload rises → size of LV increases → less obstruction
  - Murmur **DECREASES** in intensity

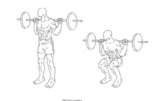

Wikipedia

HCM
Other maneuvers

- Raising the legs
  - Increases venous return
  - More VR → More preload → Bigger LV cavity
  - This moves the obstructing septum out of the way
  - Murmur **DECREASES** in intensity
- Standing
  - Opposite mechanism of leg raise
  - Murmur **INCREASES** in intensity

Aortic Stenosis

- Both HCM and AS cause a systolic ejection murmur
- Less effect of maneuvers on aortic stenosis
  - Fixed obstruction
- Opposite effects of maneuvers in aortic stenosis
  - Less preload → less flow → quieter AS murmur

HCM
Maneuver Summary

- Valsalva → INCREASE
- Standing → INCREASE
- Squatting → DECREASE
- Leg Raise → DECREASE

HCM
Associations

- **Maternal diabetes**
  - Infants: transient hypertrophic cardiomyopathy
  - Usually thickening of interventricular septum
  - May have small LV chamber → obstruction in newborn
  - Resolves by a few months of age

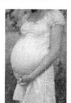

HCM
Associations

- **Friedreich Ataxia**
  - Autosomal recessive CNS disease
  - Trinucleotide repeat disorder
  - Spinocerebellar symptoms
  - Often have concentric left ventricular hypertrophy
  - Also septal hypertrophy

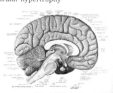

Cardiac Hypertrophy
Other Causes

- Hypertension
- Valve disease
- Athlete's heart

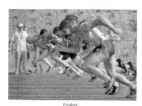

Cardiac Hypertrophy
Rare Pathologic Causes

- **Fabry Disease**
  - Lysosomal storage disease
  - Deficiency of α-galactosidase A
  - Neuropathy, skin lesions, lack of sweat
  - Left ventricular hypertrophy

Cardiac Hypertrophy
Rare Pathologic Causes

- **Pompe Disease**
  - Glycogen storage disease (develops in infancy)
  - Acid alpha-glucosidase deficiency
  - Enlarged muscles, hypotonia
  - Cardiac enlargement

Endocarditis

Jason Ryan, MD, MPH

Endocarditis

- Inflammation of endocardium of heart
- Usually involves cardiac valves
- Often causes new regurgitation murmur
- Consequence of bacteremia

Endocarditis
Echocardiogram

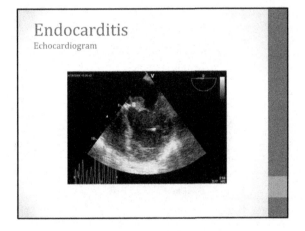

General Symptoms

- Fever
- Chills
- Sweats
- Petechiae
  - Small vessel inflammation
  - Leakage of blood

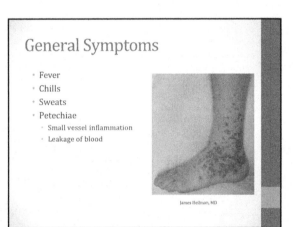

James Hellman, MD

Regurgitant Valve Disease

- Aortic regurgitation
- Mitral regurgitation
- Tricuspid regurgitation

Embolic Symptoms

- Brain (stroke)
- Spinal cord (paralysis)
- Eye (blindness)
- Legs (ischemia)
- Splenic or renal infarction
- Pulmonary embolism (tricuspid)
- Coronary artery (acute myocardial infarction)

Endocarditis Stigmata

- Physical exam findings in endocarditis
- Caused by septic emboli and immune complexes
- Very rare in modern era

Endocarditis Stigmata

- Roth spots
  - **Retinal lesions**
  - Red with pale center
- Osler nodes
  - Painful bumps on pads of fingers and toes
- Janeway lesions
  - Nontender red macules on palms and soles
- Splinter hemorrhages
  - Reddish-brown lines under fingernails

Diagnosis

- Major Duke Criteria
  - Positive blood cultures
  - Vegetation on echocardiogram
- Minor Criteria
  - Fever
  - Risk factors
  - Roth spots, Osler nodes, Janeway lesions, splinters
- 2 major, 1 major 3 minor, or 5 minor

Microbiology

- Staphylococcus aureus
- Viridans streptococcus
- Streptococcus Bovis
- Enterococcus
- Staphylococcus epidermidis
- Culture negative endocarditis
- Libman-Sacks

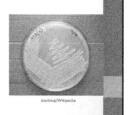

Staph Aureus

- Gram positive cocci
- Catalase positive
- Coagulase positive
- May infect **tricuspid valve in IV drug users**

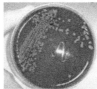

Iqbal Osman/Flikr

Staph Aureus

- Causes **acute** endocarditis
- Rapid, severe infection
- Symptoms occur over days
- Can occur in patients with **normal heart valves**
  - No pre-disposing valvular heart condition

Viridans Streptococcus

- Group of gram positive cocci
  - S. mitis, S. mutans, S. sanguinis
- Catalase negative
- Mouth flora
- Endocarditis may occur after **dental procedure**

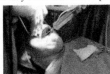

Viridans Streptococcus

- Low virulence bacteria
- Often affect **damaged valves**
  - Bacteria synthesize dextran
  - Dextran adheres to fibrin
  - Fibrin found with endothelial damage
- Classic predisposing condition: mitral valve prolapse

Viridans Streptococcus

- Causes **subacute** endocarditis
- Less severe symptoms
- Symptoms occur over days to weeks

Streptococcus Bovis

- Gram positive cocci
- Lancefield group D
- Normal gut bacteria
- Associated with **colon cancer**
  - All subtypes associated with cancer
  - Strongest association: S. gallolyticus (S. bovis type 1)

Enterococcus Endocarditis

- Gram positive cocci
- Lancefield group D
- Normal gut bacteria
- Usually a subacute endocarditis course
- Commonly occurs in **older men**
- Associated with manipulation of GI/GU tract
  - Abdominal surgery
  - Urinary catheter
  - TURP for treatment of BPH

Prosthetic Valve Endocarditis

- Occurs with mechanical or biologic valves
- Rarely cured with antibiotics
- Usually requires repeat valve surgery
- Similar bacteria to native valve endocarditis
- **Staphylococcus epidermidis**
  - Rarely cause endocarditis except in prosthetic valves

Staphylococcus Epidermidis

- Catalase positive
- Coagulase negative (unlike S. Aureus)
- Most common coagulase negative staphylococcus
- **Normal skin flora**
- Low virulence
- Commonly cause infection of prosthetic material
  - Cardiac valves
  - Intravascular catheters
  - Prosthetic joints

Culture Negative Endocarditis

- Evidence of endocarditis with sterile blood cultures
- Caused by rare bacteria difficult to culture
- Coxiella burnetii
- Bartonella

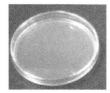
Y tambe/Wikipedia

Coxiella Burnetii

- Zoonotic bacteria (transferred from animals)
- Obligate intracellular bacteria
- Found in farm animals
- Cattle, sheep and goats
  - Abortions in farm animals: Coxiella **placenta** infection
- Humans inhale aerosolized bacteria from animals
- Causes Q fever

Coxiella Burnetii

- Acute Q fever
  - Flu-like illness
  - May present as pneumonia
  - More than half of cases: no symptoms
- Chronic Q fever
  - Most common manifestation is endocarditis

Bartonella

- Bartonella quintana
  - Small, gram-negative rod
  - Transmitted by lice
  - Patients with poor hygiene
- Bartonella henselae
  - Found in cats
  - Causes cat scratch fever

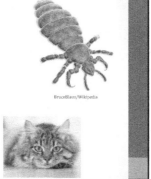
BruceBlaus/Wikipedia
Inge Wallumrød/Pexels.com

NBTE
Non-bacterial, thrombotic endocarditis

- Libman-Sacks Endocarditis or Marantic endocarditis
- Lesions on valves that look like endocarditis
- Found on **both sides of valve**
- Mitral valve most common
- Formed by thrombus, immune complexes
- Seen in hypercoagulable states
  - Advanced malignancy
  - Systemic lupus erythematosus

NBTE
Non-bacterial, thrombotic endocarditis

- Often asymptomatic identified at autopsy
- Rarely cause regurgitation or murmurs
- Thrombus easily dislodges → **embolization**
- Most patients asymptomatic until embolism occurs
- May embolize to spleen, kidney, skin, extremities
- May cause stroke
- Can cause myocardial infarction

Bacterial Endocarditis
Treatment

- Several weeks appropriate antibiotics
- Broad spectrum antibiotics initially
- Drug therapy changes when bacteria identified
- Valve surgery sometimes required
  - Large vegetation
  - Severe valve disease → heart failure

Bacterial Endocarditis
Complications

- May form abscess beneath valve annulus
- Persistent fever, bacteremia often indicates abscess
- Aortic valve abscess can lead to heart block
  - AV node dysfunction

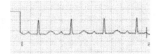

Prophylaxis

- Primary prevention for bacterial endocarditis
- Done before high-risk medical procedures
- Antibiotics given to some high-risk patients
- New guidelines restrict to highest risk circumstances

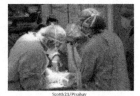
Scooth23/Pixabay

Prophylaxis

Conditions	Procedures
Prosthetic valves Prior endocarditis Cyanotic congenital heart disease Heart transplants	Dental work Respiratory procedures Skin surgery

Amoxicillin
Clindamycin

Made in the USA
Middletown, DE
15 August 2019